CONTROLLED RELEASE
OF BIOLOGICALLY
ACTIVE AGENTS

ADVANCES IN EXPERIMENTAL MEDICINE AND BIOLOGY

Recent Volumes in this Series

CONTROLLED RELEASE OF BIOLOGICALLY ACTIVE AGENTS

Edited by

A. C. Tanquary and R. E. Lacey

Southern Research Institute
Birmingham, Alabama

PLENUM PRESS • NEW YORK AND LONDON

Library of Congress Cataloging in Publication Data

Main entry under title:

Controlled release of biologically active agents.

(Advances in experimental medicine and biology, v. 47)
Proceedings of a symposium held in Birmingham, Ala., Apr. 19-20, 1973, spon-
sored by the Southern Research Institute.
Includes bibliographical references.
1. Delayed-action preparations — Congresses. I. Tanquary, A. C. II. Lacey,
Robert E., ed. III. Southern Research Institute, Birmingham, Ala. IV. Series.
[DNLM: 1. Biopharmaceutics — Congresses. 2. Delayed-action preparations —
Congresses. W1AD559 v. 47 1973 / QV38 S986c 1973]
RS201.D4C66   615'.7'04   74-8215
ISBN 0-306-39047-7

Proceedings of a Symposium held in Birmingham, Alabama,
April 19 and 20, 1973 under sponsorship of Southern
Research Institute

© 1974 Plenum Press, New York
A Division of Plenum Publishing Corporation
227 West 17th Street, New York, N.Y. 10011

United Kingdom edition published by Plenum Press, London
A Division of Plenum Publishing Company, Ltd.
4a Lower John Street, London W1R 3PD, England

Printed in the United States of America

PREFACE

The Symposium on Controlled Release of Biologically
Active Agents was held under sponsorship of Southern
Research Institute in Birmingham, Alabama, April 19 and
20, 1973. The announced purpose of the symposium was
to encourage an exchange of information among the ex-
perts working in various fields of controlled release
and the scientists and technologists interested in
applying the concepts. The number of registrants
(over 120), the diverse nature of the organizations
represented, and the enthusiastic participation of
attendees in the discussions testified to intense and
broad interests in controlled release. The papers presented at the symposium should serve well to introduce
the principles of controlled release and demonstrate a
few of the promising applications.

Controlled release is an important step toward improving the delivery of a biologically active agent to
its target. Precise administration of an agent can
substantially reduce the concentration required for
beneficial effects and thus minimize deleterious effects
to the organism or to the environment. Through controlled release, older agents whose efficacies are
established may prove more reliable, and newer agents
whose high potencies or low stabilities have inhibited
use may prove more suitable. Controlled release therefore offers both an alternative and a complementary
route to the increasingly costly and demanding search
for agents of greater specificity.

The papers in this book appear in the order of their
presentation at the symposium. The papers may not be
identical to the ones presented at the meeting, however,
because some of the papers had been condensed by speak-
ers to fit the time allotted, and some of the manuscripts
were changed by authors to clarify statements or answer
questions raised in the meeting. Moreover, we chose to
alter some of the symbols and equations to improve

clarity, especially where these had been used to express
diverse meanings.

    We are indebted to all of the authors for their co-
operation in adhering to rigid manuscript specifications,
and also to Mrs. W. Schulman for her untiring efforts in
assisting us in our editorial endeavors.

                                A. C. Tanquary
                                R. E. Lacey

Birmingham, Alabama
March 18, 1974

LIST OF CONTRIBUTORS

M. K. Akkapeddi, Polysciences, Inc., Warrington,
    Pennsylvania
G. Graham Allan, University of Washington, Seattle,
    Washington
R. W. Baker, ALZA Corporation, Palo Alto, California
H. Balin, Hahneman Medical College and Hospital,
    Philadelphia, Pennsylvania
David R. Blake, University of Maryland, Baltimore,
    Maryland
Donald R. Cowsar, Southern Research Institute,
    Birmingham, Alabama
R. H. Davis, Hahneman Medical College and Hospital,
    Philadelphia, Pennsylvania
John Eldridge, University of Delaware, Newark, Delaware
Gordon L. Flynn, University of Michigan, Ann Arbor,
    Michigan
B. D. Halpern, Polysciences, Inc., Warrington,
    Pennsylvania
Robert E. Lacey, Southern Research Institute,
    Birmingham, Alabama
Thomas Leafe, University of Delaware, Newark, Delaware
H. K. Lonsdale, Bend, Oregon
Francis Meyer, University of Maryland, Baltimore,
    Maryland
Amar Nath Neogi, University of Washington, Seattle,
    Washington
E. S. Nuwayser, Abcor, Inc., Cambridge, Massachusetts
Theodore J. Roseman, The Upjohn Company, Kalamazoo,
    Michigan
D. L. Williams, Abcor, Inc., Cambridge, Massachusetts
J. H. R. Woodland, University of Delaware, Newark,
    Delaware
S. Yolles, University of Delaware, Newark, Delaware

CONTENTS

LIST OF SYMBOLS*

A   surface area (cm^2)

B   number of chain ends per unit volume (cm^{-3})

C   concentration (g cm^{-3})

C_s solubility (g cm^{-3})

D   diffusion coefficient (diffusivity)(cm^2 sec^{-1})

F   fraction of agent released

J   flux (g cm^{-2} sec^{-1})

K   partition (distribution) coefficient

M   total mass of agent in device (g)

M_t mass of agent released at time t (g)

M_∞ mass of agent released at time t_∞ (g)

P   permeability (DK)(cm^2 sec^{-1})

Q_t mass of agent released per unit area at time
            t(M_t/A)(g cm^{-2})

R_t total diffusional resistance (cm sec)

R_a diffusional resistance of water (cm sec)

R_m diffusional resistance of matrix (cm sec)

R_s diffusional resistance of solvent (cm sec)

T   temperature (°C or °K as specified)

T_g glass-transition temperature (°K)

T_m melt temperature (°K)

*The CGS units express dimensions, not necessarily
 specific usage: for example, release rates may be
 given in µg day^{-1}, rather than g sec^{-1}.

V	volume (cm^3)
V_c	volume of matrix (continuum)(cm^3)
V_f	volume of filler (cm^3)
V_r	volume of receiving fluid (cm^3)
V_s	volume of source (cm^3)
W	mass per unit volume (M/V)($g\ cm^{-3}$)
h,ℓ	thickness of membrane (cm)
r	radius (cm)
r_i	inner radius (cm)
r_o	outer radius (cm)
t	time (sec)
$t_{\frac{1}{2}}$	half-time of exhaustion (sec)
t_∞	time of exhaustion (sec)
x	distance from membrane surface (cm)
γ	normalizing parameter (J/C_sD)(cm^{-1})
δ	jump distance (cm)
ε	porosity of matrix
λ	thickness of stagnant fluid boundary layer (cm)
ϕ	frequency of jump (sec^{-1})
τ	tortuosity of matrix

Combined Symbols

dM_t/dt	release rate ($g\ sec^{-1}$)
dQ/dt	flux (J)($g\ cm^{-2}\ sec^{-1}$)

INTRODUCTION TO CONTROLLED RELEASE

Donald R. Cowsar

Southern Research Institute

Birmingham, Alabama 35205

Scientists today, more than ever before, are being
challenged to provide new, safer, more economical, and
more efficient means of providing for the health and
well-being of mankind. In almost every instance, the
key to meeting these challenges lies in the development
of ever more ingenious methods for manipulating biological factors. Historically, scientists have dealt with
these problems by designing new biologically active
agents. However, whether these agents are pharmaceuticals or agricultural chemicals, use of these agents to
produce the desired biological responses is yet fraught
with gross inefficiencies that result primarily from
inabilities to deliver the agents to their targets
(organisms or organs) at the precise time and in the
precise quantities required. The results of these inefficiencies are obvious: the use of the agents is
costly, and undesirable side-effects (sometimes cata-
strophic in nature) occur.

To minimize side-effects, scientists have generally
concentrated on designing agents having greater specificity and less persistence. However, through a per-
verse law of nature applying to the design of agents,
the less persistent and more specific agents are almost
always costly and difficult to administer. The increased difficulties in administering the agents are
usually a consequence of labile linkages, since greater
potency with minimal persistence or side-effects usually
comes from rapid metabolism. And rapid metabolism, in

turn, means effectiveness only within narrow limits of
time and concentration. The added costs are usually a
result of both the expense of synthesis (since more
specific agents tend to be more complex) and the expense
of repeated applications.

Recognizing these limitations in the design of agents,
scientists are increasingly turning to an alternative
approach, that of improving the delivery of the agents,
both newer agents and old. This approach is soundly
based on the premise that the optimum biological response
occurs when the level and time of the availability of the
biologically active agent to the target (organism or
organ) are optimized. Agent availability is the relationship between the rate of delivery of the agent and the
rate of removal of the agent. Removal of the agents
means metabolism, chemical decomposition, deactivation,
excretion, or other methods by which agents become
inactive.

I. CONVENTIONAL AGENT DELIVERY

The designers of biologically active agents expend
vast efforts and funds synthesizing, screening, and
testing agents. However, once a promising agent has
been identified, considerably less effort is usually
spent developing the delivery system (i.e., formulating
the final dosage form). Standard criteria are usually
followed to determine the site of application or route
of administration, the unit dose or level of application,
and the most convenient application or dosage schedule.
In order to understand the importance of the role that
delivery plays in our ability to obtain optimum biological response, we should first review the shortcomings
of the delivery of agents by conventional techniques.

Agents are usually delivered systemically or topi-
cally often at a site somewhat remote from the target
(organism or organ). Figure 1 shows schematically the
delivery of an agent by conventional techniques. The
agent is administered to the biological environment
from an appropriate formulation. Route 1 in the figure
illustrates the case of "indirect" agent application
such as the oral administration of pharmaceuticals or
the application of systemic insecticides to the soil to
control insects in plants. In this case the agent first
enters a reservoir (the digestive tract or ground water)
having a volume, V_1. Here the agent becomes diluted.

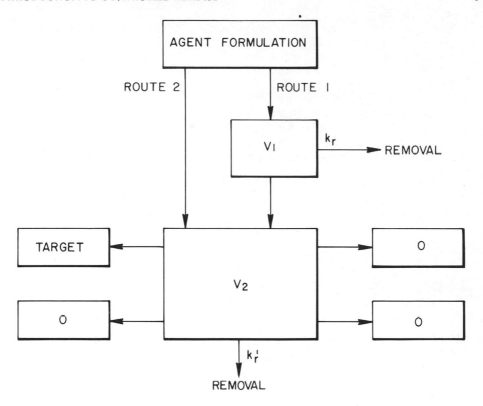

Figure 1.   Conventional Agent Delivery

Over a period of time the agent either diffuses into the
desired systemic environment (the circulatory system or
the plant sap) having volume V_2, or is removed from the
site _via_ excretion, metabolism, or chemical deactivation. In the figure, k_r is the rate constant for the
rate of removal of the agent from V_1. As the agent
enters V_2 it becomes further diluted as it is distributed
to the various organs or organisms, O, at least one of
which is the target for the agent. The action of the
agent on organs or organisms other than the target may
result in undesirable side effects. Finally, the agent
is metabolized or otherwise irreversibly removed from
V_2 at a rate governed by the removal rate constant, k_r'.
Route 2 in the figure illustrates a more direct application such as by the intravenous injection of pharmaceuticals or the spraying of crops with pesticides. The first
reservoir, V_1, is by-passed in the scheme, but side effects resulting from agent in V_2 affecting non-target
organisms or organs can still occur.

When agent is delivered by one of these conventional
routes, the level and time of availability of agent to
the target cannot be controlled independently. Only the
level and frequency of application can be manipulated.
The rate of removal of the agent from the biological
environment is usually considered to be an "uncontrol-
lable" parameter. At best, the removal of agent can be
described by typical reaction kinetics with most biological removal systems being first order or pseudo-first
order in agent concentration.

The first-order rate law states that the instanta-
neous rate of removal is proportional to the amount of
agent present. If M/V_2 is the concentration of agent
present, the rate of removal, $\frac{d(M/V_2)}{dt}$, of agent can
be expressed as

$$\frac{d(M/V_2)}{dt} = k_r(M/V_2) \tag{1}$$

where k_r is the rate constant for removal. The integrated solution to Equation (1) is

$$\ln M/M_o = k_r t \tag{2}$$

where M_o is the amount present at t=0; M_o is thus the
amount applied. The rate of removal of the agent from
the biological environment is often expressed as the
agent half-life, $t_{1/2}$. The half-life is related to the
first-order rate constant for removal as follows:

$$\ln 2 = k_r t_{1/2} \tag{3}$$

$$\text{or,} \quad k_r = \ln 2/t_{1/2} = 0.693/t_{1/2} \tag{4}$$

The magnitude of the effect that agent removal has on
agent availability can best be illustrated by examples.

Example I. Consider a pharmaceutical agent (drug)
designed to combat an infectuous disease and known by
pharmacodynamic and toxicological studies to be effective at an optimum systemic level of 5±2 µg/kg (i.e.,
at levels below 3 µg/kg the drug is only marginally
effective, and at levels above 7 µg/kg it may cause
undesirable side effects). Assume further that the
drug cannot be administered orally, that the half-life
for removal in vivo has been determined to be 8 hr, and
that patient should be treated for 10 to 14 days.

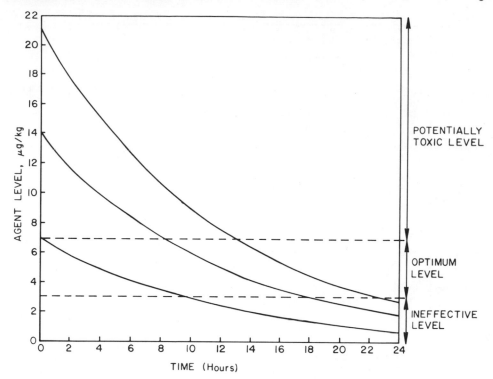

Figure 2.   Level and Duration of Agent Availability
              after Single Injection

Using Equation (4) we can calculate a pseudo-first-
order rate constant for drug removal to be 0.0866 hr^{-1}.
We can generate the drug availability profile for various dosage levels by applying Equation (2) in the exponential form,

$$M = M_o e^{-k_r t} \tag{5}$$

Figure 2 shows the levels and durations that can be
achieved by single injections of 7, 14, and 21 µg/kg of
the drug. A single injection of a 7 µg/kg dose of the
drug would obviously provide an effective drug level
for about 10 hr.   Thirty-two subsequent injections of
5 µg/kg doses at 10 hr intervals would give the desired effect. If dosages of 14 µg/kg were given to
reduce the number of needed injections, an effective
level could be maintained for about 18 hr, but for 8
hr the concentration of drug is at a hazardous level.
If single daily injections were tried, a level of 21

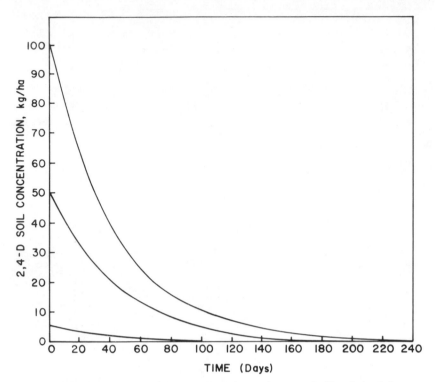

Figure 3. Level and Duration of Herbicide
Availability after a Single Application

μg/kg (three times the maximum safe level) would be
required. An injected dose that would provide an
effective level of the drug for 48 hr can be calculated
to be 192 μg/kg or approximately 30 times the safe dose.
In actual use, the drug would probably be given <u>via</u> injection every 12 hr at about 7 μg/kg per injection. This
would probably require hospitalization of the patient.

    <u>Example II</u>. Consider the use of the herbicide 2,4-D
to control weeds along highway rights-of-way in the South.
The surface soil concentration must be maintained at or
above 0.5 kg/ha for 240 days to be effective. The half-
life of 2,4-D in warm moist soil is of the order of 30
days.

    Again, we can calculate a pseudo-first-order rate
constant for removal to be k_r = 0.0231 day^{-1}. We can
generate the herbicide availability profile for various
levels of application by applying Equation (5). Figure
3 shows the level and duration of 2,4-D herbicide after

single applications of 5, 50, and 100 kg/ha to the soil.
It is apparent in the figure that application of 2,4-D
at a level of 5 kg/ha (ten times the effective level of
0.5 kg/ha) would provide protection against weeds for
approximately 100 days; application at a level of 50
kg/ha (100 times the effective level) would provide
protection for about 200 days; and a single application
at a level of 100 kg/ha (200 times the minimal effective
level) would be required to obtain protection for 240
days.

To summarize, the delivery of agents by conventional
techniques can be grossly inefficient. Whether measured
in gallons or kilograms or milliliters or micrograms,
vast amounts of agents are employed where smaller amounts
would be thought to suffice. The use of large amounts
of agents in single applications greatly increases the
incidence of undesirable side effects because non-target
organisms or organs are swamped with potentially toxic
agents to ensure that the target will receive an effective dose for the desired period of time. When agent
applications (dosages) are divided to increase efficiency,
lesser amounts of agents are effective but frequent applications can be very costly.

II.   CONTROLLED DELIVERY

If one attempts to optimize conventional agent delivery to maximize agent availability with a minimum
amount of the agent, one finds that the repeated application of small increments of the total dose will, in
theory, produce the desired effect. For pharmaceuticals this means continuous infusions of the drugs and
for agricultural chemicals this means daily applications
of the agents. Obviously, incremental or continuous applications of agents by conventional agent delivery systems are impossible or impractical. However, the method
becomes practical and indeed highly promising when one
considers the possibility of a new type of dosage form
consisting of a protected supply of agent from which the
agent is automatically released at a controlled rate over
a long period of time.

Figure 4 schematically shows the concept of controlled
release of biologically active agents. The figure has
some obvious similarities with Figure 1 which depicts
conventional agent delivery. For controlled release,
however, the delivery rate constants, k_d, are important

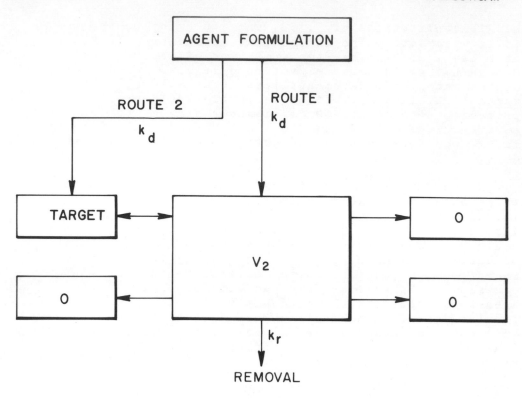

Figure 4.   Controlled Delivery
of Agents

parts of the delivery scheme. For delivery via "Route 1",
a controlled-release formulation of the agent is administered to the total systemic biological environment by a
conventional method (i.e., injection, implantation,
spreading, or spraying). The formulation is an agent
reservoir that protects the stored agent from removal
mechanisms and delivers the agent to the biological
reservoir, V_2, at a predetermined (programmed) rate, k_d.
Only the released agent is subject to removal systems
(metabolism, excretion, etc.). For delivery via "Route
2", the controlled release formulation is positioned in
the biological environment in close proximity to the
target (organ or organism) to permit delivery of the
agent directly to the target at a rate, k_d. For agent
delivery via Route 1 the total volume, V_2 (or area or
mass), of the systemic environment is still an important
variable since, like in conventional delivery, the released agent is diluted by this V_2 factor. For agent

delivery _via_ Route 2, however, very little dilution
occurs and, hence, even smaller amounts of agent are
required to produce the optimum biological response.

The kinetics of removal of the agent from the biological environment are usually independent of the
dosage form or delivery system. Thus, the half-life and
rate constant, k_r, for the removal of the released agent
are the same as for conventional systemic delivery systems. The level and time of agent availability, however,
are not functions of the removal rate and the total
amount of agent in the dosage form, but rather are functions of the removal rate and the rate of release of
the agent from the delivery system. The rate of release of agent from a controlled-release dosage form
depends upon a number of factors which will be discussed
in detail in subsequent chapters. If the agent is delivered at a constant rate (zero-order kinetics), the
delivery rate can be expressed mathematically as

$$\frac{dM}{dt} = k_d \qquad\qquad (6)$$

If the agent removal follows pseudo-first-order kinetics
where the rate of removal is

$$\frac{dM}{dt} = k_r M, \qquad\qquad (7)$$

then the level of agent availability will be constant
when the rate of delivery equals the rate of removal,
or when

$$k_d - k_r M \qquad\qquad (8)$$

The level of agent availability will be

$$M = k_d/k_r \qquad\qquad (9)$$

In the case of Example I discussed previously, the
drug had a value of k_r = 0.0866 hr^{-1}. A controlled-
release dosage form that delivers the drug _via_ Route 1
(say intramuscularly) at a constant rate, k_d, of 0.433
µg/kg hr^{-1} would maintain the systemic level of the drug
at 5 µg/kg, the optimum level. The total amount of drug
required to maintain that level for 14 days would be
approximately 110 µg/kg (or about 8 mg for a 75 kg
patient). This can be compared to a total dose of about
15 mg when the drug is administered in 7 µg/kg doses

every 12 hr. If the infection were localized and the
drug could be administered in a controlled-release
formulation at the site of infection (i.e., via Route 2)
a total dose equal to the unit dose or 0.11 mg would
probably be sufficient.

In the case of 2,4-D discussed in Example II previously, since the value of k_r was 0.0231 day^{-1}, a controlled-release formulation that has a delivery rate,
k_d, of 0.0125 kg/ha day^{-1} would maintain the soil concentration of 2,4-D at an effective level of above 0.5
kg/ha. The total amount of herbicide required for 240
days of protection would be 3.5 kg/ha via controlled
release compared to 100 kg/ha via a single conventional
application.

Controlled release is not synonymous with slow release, a much older and well recognized concept from
which the new science is emerging, although the two are
similar in principle and sometimes overlap. Slow-release
formulations are so-called because they contain several
times the normal single dose and they provide for replacement of agent at some rate which gives a measurable increase in the length of time activity. The rate may
decrease due to gradual loss of agent, or increase
through a maximum due to breakdown of a protective barrier. A controlled-release formulation, in contrast,
may exhibit a fast or a slow release, or a constant or
a changing release, depending on the design. The principle difference lies not entirely in the profiles of
release but in the mechanism of release. The distinction is drawn mainly by the degree of control of both
the optimum level and the optimum time of availability
of the biologically active agent.

III.   CONTROLLED-RELEASE FORMULATIONS
AND DELIVERY SYSTEMS

In the context of the current state-of-the-art, a
controlled-release formulation or delivery system is a
combination of biologically active agent and excipient,
commonly a polymeric material, arranged to allow delivery of the agent to the target (organ or organism)
at controlled rates over a specified period of time.
Many design variations of these systems have been
studied or proposed. Seven of these are the following:
(1) capsules of polymeric material filled with a solid
or liquid agent or with a suspension or solution of

agent in a fluid, in which the release of agent is controlled by Fickian diffusion through the capsule walls;
(2) a heterogeneous dispersion of particles of agent in
a solid polymeric matrix, which can be either biodegradable or non-biodegradable and which controls the
release of agent by diffusion through the matrix, by
erosion of the matrix, or by a combination of both diffusion and erosion; (3) a laminate of agent and polymeric
material made by coating a film of biodegradable or non-
biodegradable material with solid agent and then forming
the film into a sealed "sandwich" or "jelly roll", which
controls release of agent by diffusion, by erosion, or
by both; (4) a heterogeneous dispersion or solution of
agent in a water-swellable hydrogel matrix, which controls release of the agent by slow surface-to-center
swelling of the matrix by water and consequent diffusion of the agent from the water-swollen part of the
matrix; (5) liquid-liquid encapsulation of the agent in
a viscous solution ("syrup") of polymer, which controls
release of agent by slow diffusion through or dilution
of the media; (6) chemical bonding of the agent to a
polymeric backbone, as by pendant amide or ester linkages, which controls release of the agent by hydrolysis;
and (7) formation of macromolecular structures of the
agent via ionic or covalent linkages, which controls
release of the agent by hydrolysis, thermodynamic dis-
sociation or microbial degradation of the linkages. In
most of the systems now being studied, the rate of release of the agent is controlled primarily by diffusion
through a polymeric membrane.

The designers of controlled-release formulations or
delivery systems must have an unusually high degree of
understanding of a variety of design parameters and system variables in order to develop the desired degree of
control. Because of the magnitude and interdisciplinary
nature of the effort, the task cannot be undertaken
lightly, but must be fully justified by the increased
value of the system. Dosage-form design cannot be mere-
ly appended to an extensive agent development program.
In fact, in the context of current FDA regulations, most
agent-excipient controlled-release formulations are considered new drugs and must be subjected to extensive
safety and efficacy evaluations even if the components
have been separately approved.

Some of the factors that must be considered by designers of controlled-release systems are the following: (1) The optimum level of agent necessary to obtain

the desired biological response. (For controlled-release
systems this level is almost always much lower than the
level required for application by conventional techniques.) (2) The mechanisms and rates of all agent removal systems operable in the biological environment.
(These include agent metabolism, excretion, and deactivation. A first-order rate law was assumed here--actual
rate laws will affect the results to the extent that
they differ.) (3) The kinetics and mechanism of the
delivery of agent from the release system chosen. (This
is the subject of several chapters of this publication.)
(4) The influence of the biological environment on the
mechanism and kinetics of release. (Since most controlled-release systems are agent-polymer combinations
and since the properties of most polymers are affected
by prolonged exposure to the elements of agricultural
and physiological environments, one must be aware of
possible changes and allow for them. It can generally
be said that a satisfactory controlled-release formulation or device should be practically independent of the
changeable conditions that exist in the biological environment.) (5) Inherent restrictions on the physical
and chemical properties of the delivery system materials
dictated by the particular application. (These include
such limitations as reversibility, biodegradability, and
acceptability of residues.)

IV. APPLICATIONS

The number of applications that have been or can be
visualized for controlled-release formulations is immense. Current commercialized applications are few but
a number of systems are in the research and development
stage. Insecticide strips and flea-collars are now
familiar consumer items. Controlled-release herbicides
and fertilizer formulations are being test marketed in
some sections of the country. Alza Corporation, a
pioneer in this field, is demonstrating in clinical
trials that intrauterine devices that release progesterone at low constant rates can be effective for contraception for a year or more. The Alza IUD's contain
the equivalent dosage of three oral pills and the
amount released daily is low enough not to interrupt
the normal menstrual cycle. Side effects are thus
minimal. Even further along in development is another
Alza controlled-release device called an Ocusert. When
inserted in the cul-de-sac of the eye, the device de-

livers a minimal therapeutic dose of pilocarpine to the eye continuously for a week, thus attenuating the effects of glaucoma.

Today's high cost of beef is at least partially due to inefficient supply. A controlled-release device for syncronizing estrous cycles in beef cattle could greatly improve the efficacy of artificial insemination programs, so that cattle farms, which are becoming beef factories, could produce calves on schedule and thus become more completely mechanized. Searle Laboratories, and possibly others, are currently perfecting delivery systems for steroidal hormones that can regulate estrus in cattle.

Some of the other agents and applications that are being researched include delivery systems for antimalarial agents, anticancer drugs, narcotic antagonists, abortifacients, algaecides, insect hormones and pheromones, insecticides, and plant nutrients. The ultimate goal of pharmaceutical controlled-release systems may well be an implantable device that releases agent on physiological demand. An "artificial pancreas", which releases insulin in response to high blood-sugar levels, is one of the devices now being researched by several groups. The current approach involves the development of a small implantable glucose-sensing olootrode that can be coupled through a miniature computer logic system to a refillable implanted insulin infusion pump.

It should be pointed out that many agents are not amenable to administration by controlled-release formulations or devices, and other agents can be delivered equally effectively by simple alternative means. Nevertherless, the new technology provides fresh sound approaches to overcoming inefficient delivery of most biologically active agents, long a barrier to the fuller utilization of these materials.

CONTROLLED RELEASE: MECHANISMS AND RATES

R. W. Baker
ALZA Corporation
Palo Alto, California   93404
    and
H. K. Lonsdale
Route 3, Box 1352
Bend, Oregon   97701

I.   INTRODUCTION

Historical

In its broadest sense, the concept of sustained or prolonged release of beneficial agents has been in existence for decades. The earliest commercial applications of this concept apparently occurred in the agricultural[1,2] and pharmaceutical industries.[3-5] In agriculture, slow-release fertilizers have been in use for more than 25 years. The methods include use of compounds of low water solubility, and hence low dissolution rates; use of nitrogenous compounds that are slowly activated by microbial action; membrane-regulated devices in which a membrane surrounds the fertilizer which is released by diffusion through the membrane, or erosion of the membrane; and complexation of the active component with, for example, ion-exchange resins.

In the pharmaceutical field, prolonged release has been widely used in oral medications since the early 1950's. The history of this application, as well as the technology, advantages, and limitations, has been reviewed.[3-5] The methods commonly used are similar to those cited above, namely, encapsulated pellets or beads, enteric coated formulations, slightly soluble salts, complexation, and porous tablets containing dispersed drug.

15

The 1964 report by Folkman and co-workers[6] that silicone rubber is permeable to a variety of drugs and is also
compatible with tissue encouraged several workers to de-
vise sustained-release drug delivery devices for applications other than simple oral medicaments. For example,
implantable devices have been studied for sustained release of pacemaker drugs,[6] anesthetics,[7-9] antimalarial
and antischistosomal agents,[10] atropine and histamine,[11]
and a variety of steroids for fertility control in both
women and men.[12-30] Virtually all of these studies have
involved the use of silicone rubber as the capsule material, and a nonquantitative summary of the drugs to which
this material is permeable has been presented by Folkman
and Mark.[7] Tissue reactions to silicone rubber and other
materials have been studied,[31-34] as have the effects of
osmotic pressure on implanted capsules.[35] Recently, an
externally controllable implant has been suggested,[36]
along with the use of "chemodes" or "dialytrodes" for the
perfusion of a specific locus (usually a portion of the
brain) with drugs.[37,38] The use of membrane-controlled
drug delivery devices is not limited to implants. Indeed,
this mode of use is often not preferred because it involves a surgical procedure which is not easily reversed.
Another and more preferred mode of entry to the body is
to place the device in a body cavity; for example, the
vagina, the uterus, or the cul-de-sac of the eye. An
example of this type of device is the uterine progesterone delivery system being developed at the ALZA Corporation. This device is designed to deliver a contraceptive
drug, progesterone, at the level of tens of micrograms
per day for one or more years. Another ALZA device currently undergoing Phase III clinical trials is the
pilacarpine OCUSERT® delivery system which is a membrane-
controlled device which resides in the cul-de-sac of the
eye, delivering pilocarpine at a precisely controlled
rate. With this device, glaucoma can be treated on a
continuous basis.

In this paper, our interest in controlled release
lies in the pharmaceutical field, but the same sustained-
release concepts involving encapsulation or dispersion
within release rate-controlling media are used in applications as diverse as pesticides[2,39,40] and antibacterial
plastics.[41,42]

Scope of This Paper

Let us first make the distinction between controlled
release and sustained or prolonged release. Sustained

release can be achieved by a number of methods, some of
which have already been cited: complexation, slowly dissolving coatings, use of derivatives or new compounds of
reduced solubility, and the like. In general, these
mechanisms are sensitive to the environmental conditions
to which they are exposed; e.g., the pH, motility, and
other variables along the gastrointestinal tract. In
controlled-release devices, on the other hand, the release rate is determined by the device itself. This
permits a more accurate, reproducible, and predictable
administration rate. We will be discussing only controlled-release devices. Furthermore, we will limit
ourselves to a discussion of devices involving the use of
membranes to control the release rate. Thus, the rate is
determined, in general, by the solution to Fick's laws,
with the appropriate boundary conditions.

Two types of membrane-moderated, controlled-release
devices will be described: (1) those in which the active
agent forms a core surrounded by an inert diffusion
barrier (i.e., "reservoir" devices); and (2) those in
which the active agent is dissolved or dispersed in an
inert diffusion barrier (i.e., "monolithic" devices).
Each of these devices can exist in a variety of shapes,
of course, and the release rates are presented for three
of the most common configurations: the slab, the
cylinder, and the sphere.

Results are generally presented in two ways, as release rate vs time or as fractional release vs time. The
solutions to the diffusion equations are usually given in
terms of assumed values for the relevant parameters:
device dimensions, permeability, and so on. We have tried
to select typical values but, more importantly, we have
tried to make clear how the release rate scales with
changes in the parameters so that semi-quantitative release rates can be estimated for specific devices. The
fate of the active agent after release from the device
is beyond the scope of this paper. This may involve other
diffusive or convective processes and, for biologically
active agents, this is the province of pharmacokinetics.
The problem of boundary-layer effects is discussed here
in some detail, however, because, judged from the examples
in the literature, release rates from devices in vivo are
sometimes perturbed by the presence of unstirred layers
adjacent to the device.

Many of the solutions presented here have already
appeared in the literature. These are reproduced here,
with references, along with a number of new solutions to

provide a reasonably complete set of results within the
defined scope. While the emphasis is on drug delivery,
it may be noted that these solutions are valid beyond
the confines of biologically active agents.

II. MEMBRANES

The most important class of membrane in sustained release devices is the nonporous, homogeneous polymeric film,
through which transport occurs by a process of dissolution
of the permeating species in the polymer at one interface
and diffusion down a gradient in thermodynamic activity.
These membranes are usually referred to as solution-diffusion membranes. Silicone rubber, polyethylene, and
nylon films are typical examples. Most solution-diffusion
membranes are measurably permeable to low molecular weight
permeants (M.W. <400), and many important drugs fall into
this category.

Transport through these membranes is governed by a
simple equation, namely Fick's first law:

$$J = -D \frac{dC_m}{dx} , \tag{1}$$

where J is the flux in g/cm^2-sec, C_m is the concentration
of permeant in the membrane in g/cm^3, dC_m/dx is the
gradient in concentration, and D is the diffusion coefficient of the permeant in the membrane in cm^2/sec.
The minus sign reflects the fact that the direction of
flow is down the gradient in concentration. For all
cases of interest here, the permeant on either side of
the membrane is in equilibrium with the respective surface layer of membrane, and the concentration just inside the membrane surface can then be related to the
concentration in the adjacent solution, C, by the
expressions:

$$C_{m(o)} = KC_{(o)} \text{ at the upstream surface } (x = o)$$
$$C_{m(\ell)} = KC_{(\ell)} \text{ at the downstream surface } (x = \ell). \tag{2}$$

Here, K is a distribution coefficient and is analogous to
the familiar liquid-liquid partition coefficient. A
schematic representation of the concentration profile

through a membrane is presented in Figure 1, where, for purposes of illustration, it has been assumed that the distribution coefficient is less than unity.

Throughout the following we will assume diffusion coefficients and distribution coefficients to be constant. This is a safe assumption for most polymer-drug systems because of the generally low solubility of most drugs in polymers. Thus, in the steady state, Equation (1) can be integrated to give

$$J = D \; \frac{C_m(o) - C_m(\ell)}{\ell} = D \; \frac{\Delta C_m}{\ell} \; , \tag{3}$$

where ℓ is the thickness of the membrane. Since the concentration within the membrane is usually not known, Equation (3) is frequently written

$$J = \frac{DK\Delta C}{\ell} \; , \tag{4}$$

where ΔC is the difference in concentration between the solutions on either side of the membrane.

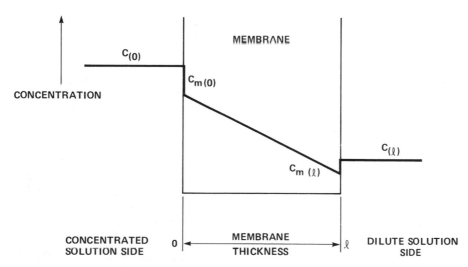

Figure 1.   Schematic representation of the concentration gradient across a membrane

Solution-Diffusion Membranes

Figure 2 illustrates some of the features of diffusion of solutes in polymers. First, diffusion in polymers is much more sensitive to molecular weight (M.W.) than is diffusion in liquids. Second, the difference in diffusion coefficient between polymers and water is relatively small for small molecules such as He and H_2, but becomes extremely large when the molecular weight reaches a few hundred. In simple terms, this is because only one or two polymer segments are involved in the movement of small molecules, but with larger molecules, several segments must be reoriented to allow the molecule to move from site to site. A cooperative movement large enough to allow this to happen is naturally relatively infrequent and the probability decreases as the molecule gets larger. Thus, the diffusion coefficients of drugs in polymers are small and decrease sharply with molecular size. Third, we can expect that polymers with relatively stiff backbones such as polystyrene will find it more difficult to undergo a large reorientation than polymers with flexible backbones, such as natural rubber, which in turn are more rigid than a liquid. Thus, the slope of the plot of log D vs log M.W. is strongly dependent on the nature of the medium. In polymers with stiff backbones, this slope can be 5 or greater, whereas in water, it is only approximately 0.5. It is interesting to note that the permeants used to generate the data in Figure 2 were not members of homologous series but were compounds of quite diverse chemistry, indicating that within a given medium the diffusion coefficient is determined principally by the size of the permeant molecule and not by its chemistry. This matter of the mass dependence of diffusion coefficients has been considered for the diffusion of gases in polymers by Michaels and Bixler[43] and for biological membranes by Stein and co-workers,[44-46] with qualitatively similar conclusions. Diffusion of solutes in polymers has been treated in greater detail elsewhere.[47,48]

Permeation rate through the membranes under consideration here is also directly proportional to the membrane/solution distribution coefficient, K. This is just the ratio of the solubility of the permeant in the polymeric membrane to that in the surrounding liquid medium. For neutral molecules, this distribution coefficient is usually independent of concentration. At this time, there are no reliable methods for quantitatively predicting the distribution coefficient, and the axiom that "like dissolves like" is still a good starting point.

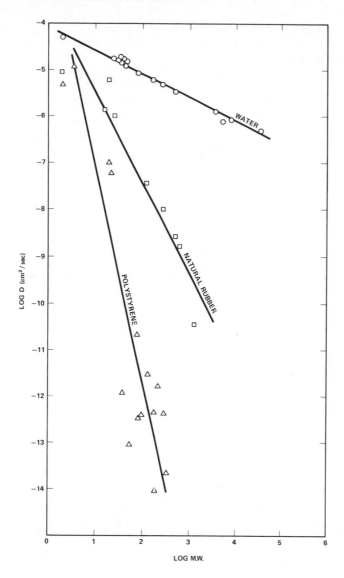

Figure 2. Plot of log D vs log M.W. for solutes diffusing in water,[49] natural rubber,[49] and polystyrene.[50-52] Diffusion coefficients of
solutes in polymers usually lie between the
value in rubber, a relatively permeable polymer, and the value in polystyrene, a relatively impermeable material. The solutes shown
in this figure are compounds of quite diverse
chemistry, namely, the gases H_2, N_2, O_2, CO_2,
etc., and halogenated paraffins in the case
of polystyrene and complex azonapthalene dyes
in the case of natural rubber.

In recent years, the solubility theory of Hildebrand has been used to develop a solubility parameter with which solubilities in liquids and polymers, liquid-liquid miscibility, and the like can be estimated. The methods have been described by Hansen,[53-55] Burrell,[56-58] and others,[59-67] and the solubility parameters of a number of polymers are now tabulated in the literature.[68]

In principle, one can thus estimate membrane permeabilities from the molecular weight of the permeant using relationships of the type shown in Figure 2 and from distribution coefficients obtained from solubility parameters. However, for solution-diffusion membranes, both of these estimates usually involve rather large uncertainties, and for the biologically-active agents of interest here, there are usually insufficient data for estimating either D or K. It is customary then to measure these permeabilities. Several such series of measurements have been carried out in recent years for solution-diffusion membranes and for a variety of drugs, and some selected values from the literature are collected in Table I for silicone rubber. Reliable permeation data for medium molecular weight species through polymers are surprisingly rare and in even fewer cases are both diffusion and distribution coefficients reported.

A few comments are in order. In this paper, we will define permeability, P, as the product of the diffusivity and the distribution coefficient. It has dimensions $(length)^2/time$, typically cm^2/sec. (It is not uncommon to find in the literature the grouping DK/ℓ [dimensions: length/time] referred to as the permeability, particularly in those cases where the membrane thickness is unknown.) The quantity J_{lim}, given in Table I, refers to the maximum steady state flux attainable (i.e., from a saturated-solution source) through a membrane 1 mm thick, Obviously, this quantity scales simply with the reciprocal of the membrane thickness. Most of the data were obtained using Dow Corning Silastic® silicone rubber membranes, which are known to contain as much as 20-30 wt% of inorganic filler material. This filler acts as an adsorbent and can affect the apparent diffusion coefficient significantly, but its effect on the permeability is generally small.[71] All the data in the table have been rounded to one significant figure accuracy; in view of the reproducibility from laboratory to laboratory (see, for example, the two results for progesterone), we feel that this is the precision the results warrant. It is important to note that the permeabilities are all based on aqueous solutions contacting the membrane. If

Table I. Selected Membrane Permeabilities and Saturated-Solution Fluxes at 37°C

Permeant	Membrane	P=DK (cm²/sec)	$J_{lim}\left(\frac{\mu g-mm}{cm^2-hr}\right)$	Source
chlormadinone acetate	unfilled silicone	2×10^{-5}	0.9	Haleblian, et al[69]
4'-aminoacetophenone	unfilled silicone	8×10^{-8}	30	Flynn and Roseman[70]
ethyl p-aminobenzoate	unfilled silicone (27°C)	2×10^{-6}	7	Most[71]
4'-aminoacetophenone	Silastic*	2×10^{-7}	20	Garrett and Chemburkar[72-73]
4'-aminopropiophenone	Silastic	5×10^{-7}	6	Garrett and Chemburkar
barbital	Silastic	3×10^{-9}	0.6	Garrett and Chemburkar
pentobarbital	Silastic	8×10^{-8}	2	Garrett and Chemburkar
phenobarbital	Silastic	1×10^{-8}	0.4	Garrett and Chemburkar
dextromethorphan	Silastic	5×10^{-6}	5	Garrett and Chemburkar
progesterone	Silastic	6×10^{-7}	0.4	Garrett and Chemburkar
caffeine	Silastic (30°C)	8×10^{-9}	6	Nakano and Patel[74]
salicylamide	Silastic (30°C)	9×10^{-8}	7	Nakano and Patel
progesterone	Silastic	8×10^{-6}	2	Kincl, et al[13-15]
testosterone	Silastic	7×10^{-6}	1	Kincl, et al
megestrol acetate	Silastic	1×10^{-5}	1	Kincl, et al
estradiol	Silastic	2×10^{-7}	0.3	Kincl, et al
cortisol	Silastic	6×10^{-9}	0.03	Kincl, et al

*Silastic® is the trade name of Dow Corning's medical grade silicone rubber.

the permeation measurements were performed in a different
medium, the permeability value would change accordingly:
D would remain unchanged but K would vary to reflect the
altered solubility in the liquid medium. The maximum
flux, J_{lim}, would remain unchanged. Permeability data
for other medium molecular weight permeant-polymer combinations can be found in the literature (see, for example,
the papers by Long,[75-77] Park,[78] Prager,[79] and their co-
workers, and the book edited by Crank and Park[47]).

A major conclusion to be drawn from Table I and
Figure 2 is that the release rates attainable from solution-diffusion membrane-controlled devices are constrained
simply because of physical limitations. Silicone rubber
is an extremely permeable polymer and yet the saturated
solution flux rarely exceeds 10 μg-mm/cm^2-hr. Since the
thinnest membranes that can be reproducibly made and
handled by conventional techniques are in the region of
50 μ, the maximum release rates obtainable with most
solution-diffusion membranes are of the order 200 μg/cm^2-
hr. Even this value is high for any polymer other than
the most flexible backbone rubbers, and with a glassy
polymer, such as polystyrene, release rates will seldom
exceed 1 μg/cm^2-hr. In addition, the value of 200 μg/cm^2-
hr for silicone rubber applies only to low and moderate
molecular weight drugs. If the molecular weight of the
drug exceeds 500 or so, we must expect a substantial decrease in achievable release rate because of the sharp
decrease in diffusion coefficient illustrated in Figure 2.

III.   THERMODYNAMICS

Fick's law, presented in Equation (1), is a phenomeno-
logical relationship which has been found experimentally
to have broad-ranging validity. However, from irrevers-
ible thermodynamics, it can be shown that the flux in
reality is proportional to the gradient in the thermodynamic activity, and Fick's law is a simplification of
the more general statement, valid because in most cases
the activity coefficient is approximately unity and concentration and activity are essentially identical. The
distinction between activity and concentration becomes
important when we have solutions of drug in different
solvents. The permeation rate through a membrane in contact with these solutions will be proportional to the
activity and not the concentration, and a solute of the
same concentration in different solvents can permeate the
membrane at widely different rates.

In designing devices that deliver at a constant rate over a prolonged period, it is essential to maintain the thermodynamic activity of the active agent within the device at some fixed value. The most convenient fixed point is unit activity, achievable by means of a saturated solution with excess solid phase present (or a pure liquid phase if the active agent is a liquid at the temperature of interest) or, simply, with only solid phase present. Unit activity and therefore constant release can then be maintained as long as excess pure solid (or liquid) phase is present.

IV.   KINETICS OF CONTROLLED RELEASE

In this section are presented steady-state and non-steady-state devices incorporating the membranes described in Section II. Several examples from the literature and the Alza Research Laboratories are presented. The importance of boundary-layer effects is also discussed.

Reservoir Devices

If a drug or other agent it enclosed within an inert membrane, and if the thermodynamic activity of the drug is maintained constant within the enclosure, then a steady state will be established during which the release rate will be constant. This is commonly referred to in the literature as "zero-order release", a term suggested by chemical kinetics. If, however, the drug is initially present within the enclosure as an undersaturated solution (or a saturated solution with no excess solid phase present), the thermodynamic activity and hence the release rate will fall exponentially. This is called "first-order release".

Constant Activity Source. The release rate of a reservoir device is determined by the membrane permeability and the device configuration. For a slab or sandwich geometry illustrated below, Fick's law can be restated:

$$\frac{dM_t}{dt} = \frac{ADK\Delta C}{\ell} \, , \tag{5}$$

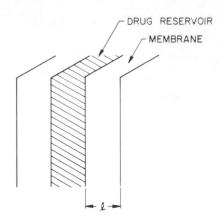

where M_t is the mass of drug released, dM_t/dt is the
steady state release rate at time t, A is the surface
area of the device (both surfaces, edge effects are
ignored), DK is the membrane permeability, and ΔC is the
difference between the internal and external drug concentration. The total amount of drug release up to any
time, t, is obtained by integrating Equation (5).

For several other geometries, the appropriate statement of Fick's law is presented in the classic texts in
the field.[80],[81] For the cylinder, the steady state release rate (ignoring end effects) is given by:

$$\frac{dM_t}{dt} = \frac{2\pi hDK\Delta C}{\ln (r_o/r_i)} \tag{6}$$

where r_o and r_i are the outside and inside radius,
respectively, and h is the length of the cylinder.

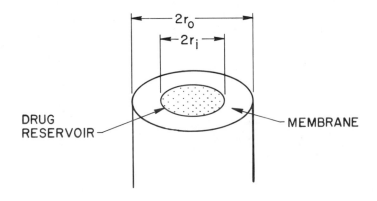

For the sphere:

$$\frac{dM_t}{dt} = 4\pi DK\Delta C \, \frac{r_o r_i}{r_o - r_i} \tag{7}$$

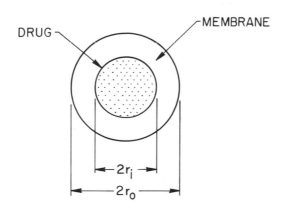

The sphere is a particularly interesting geometry since in the limit as $r_o/r_i \to \infty$, $dM_t/dt \to 4\pi DKr_i\Delta C$, i.e., the release rate becomes independent of the outer radius of the device, r_o. Figure 3 shows a plot of flux against the ratio r_o/r_i. When r_o/r_i exceeds about 4, further increases in device size for a fixed radius core do not significantly change the release rate since almost all the concentration decrease is within a distance of a few radii of the inner core. Thus, a bean-sized reservoir embedded in a golf-ball-sized matrix has the same steady-state release rate as the same core in a matrix the size of the moon (although there might be no appreciable steady state in the latter case). Furthermore, two small reservoirs placed a short distance apart on either side of the center of a sphere will have almost twice the release rate of a single reservoir, i.e., release rate in this case can be altered by the distribution and shape of the reservoirs.

Two examples of zero-order release from a constant-activity-source reservoir device are presented in Figure 4.[82] The amount of drug released from each of two sandwich-type devices is plotted against time. Both devices had essentially the same area and membrane thickness. The difference in release rate was achieved by using membranes of different permeability. In both devices the release rate was constant. In one of the devices the supply of drug in the reservoir became exhausted after which the release stopped abruptly.

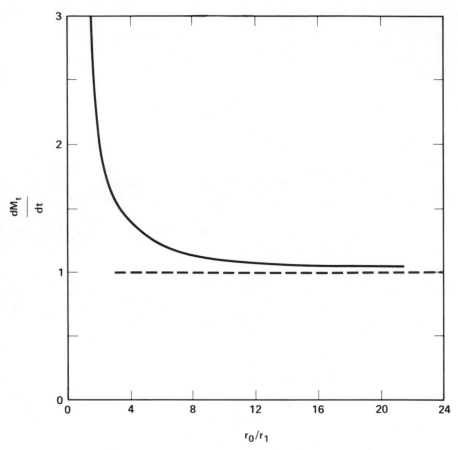

Figure 3.   A plot of release rate for a sphere containing drug at constant activity in which the
inner radius of the device is kept constant
(r_i = 1) and the outer radius (r_o) is stead-
ily increased. Once the ratio r_o/r_i exceeds
about 4, further increase in the size of the
sphere does not decrease the release rate
(Eq. 7: $4\pi DK\Delta C = 1$).

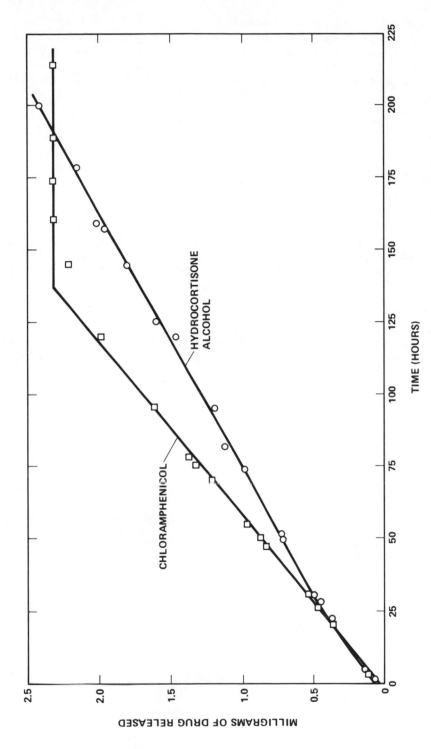

Figure 4. Drug release vs time for two constant-activity sandwich type devices.

Examples of release from spherical intrauterine devices are presented in Figure 5.[83] The cores of hollow, quarter-inch-diameter silicone rubber spheres were filled with micronized progesterone or chlormadinone acetate in a silicone rubber binder. The initial release is fairly constant, although there is a slight unaccounted for increase in release rate with time. The variation in release rate was obtained by varying the inner core radius, r_i.

Nonconstant Source. For several reasons, it may not be practical to maintain unit thermodynamic activity of the drug within the reservoir. Even in those cases where unit activity is initially established, continual loss of drug or dilution by imbibed water can eventually produce a situation where the drug activity falls with time. One example of the mathematical treatment of such problems is presented here. Extensions to several related cases should be straightforward.

Consider a reservoir of volume V_1 separated by the rate-controlling membrane from the receiving fluid, a sink of volume V_2. Let the time-dependent mass of drug in the reservoir be M_{1t} and that in the sink be M_{2t}. Then the total mass of drug, M_∞, is given by

$$M_\infty = M_{1t} + M_{2t} \;,$$

and, if all the drug is initially within the reservoir,

$$M_{1t} = M_\infty \text{ at } t = 0.$$

The concentrations and masses are related as follows:

$$M_{1t} = C_{1t}V_1$$
$$M_{2t} = C_{2t}V_2 \;.$$

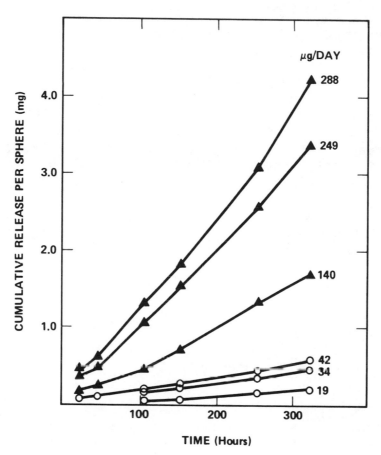

Figure 5.   *In vitro* release of chlormadinone acetate and
progesterone from spherical silicone elastomer
IUDs. ◯ Chlormadinone acetate,
▲ progesterone.[83]

32   R. W. BAKER AND H. K. LONSDALE

By use of quantities previously defined, the rate of permeation through the membrane is:

$$\frac{dM_{1t}}{dt} = - \frac{ADK}{\ell}\left(C_{1t} - C_{2t}\right) = - \frac{ADK}{\ell}\left(\frac{M_{1t}}{V_1} - \frac{M_{2t}}{V_2}\right). \tag{8}$$

Substituting for M_{2t} and rearranging,

$$\frac{dM_{1t}}{M_{1t}\left(V_2+V_1\right) - M_\infty V_1} = - \frac{ADKdt}{\ell V_1 V_2}, \tag{9}$$

This can be readily integrated, and the integration constant is evaluated by noting that $M_{1t} = M_\infty$ at t = 0. The solution is:

$$M_{1t} = \frac{M_\infty}{V_2+V_1}\left\{ V_2 \exp\left[\frac{-ADK(V_1+V_2)t}{\ell V_1 V_2}\right] + V_1\right\}. \tag{10}$$

Differentiating Equation (10) we arrive at the release rate:

$$\frac{dM_{1t}}{dt} = - \frac{M_\infty ADK}{V_1 \ell} \exp\left[\frac{-ADK(V_1+V_2)t}{\ell V_1 V_2}\right]. \tag{11}$$

Note that M_{1t} is the amount of drug remaining in the device, and not the amount released as we have used in previous examples. A useful result derivable from Equation (10) is the "half-time", $t_{\frac{1}{2}}$, or the time required to release half the drug. This is the time at which $M_{1t} = M_\infty/2$; substituting this into Equation (10) and rearranging leads to:

$$t_{\frac{1}{2}} = - \frac{\ell V_1 V_2}{ADK(V_1+V_2)} \ln\left(\frac{V_2-V_1}{2V_2}\right). \tag{12}$$

In the special case when the sink volume is very large, i.e., $V_2 >> V_1$, Equations (10), (11), and (12) become:

$$M_{1t} = M_\infty \exp\left(\frac{-ADKt}{\ell V_1}\right) ,$$ (13)

$$\frac{dM_{1t}}{dt} = -\frac{M_\infty ADK}{\ell V_1} \exp\left(\frac{-ADKt}{\ell V_1}\right),$$ (14)

$$t_{\frac{1}{2}} = -\frac{\ell V_1}{ADK} \ln(1/2) = 0.693 \frac{\ell V_1}{ADK} ,$$ (15)

respectively.

This first-order release behavior is illustrated in Figure 6 where, for simplicity, we have assumed $ADK/\ell V_1 = 1$. The important conclusions are that both the fractional release and the fractional release rate increase with increasing initial loading and fall off exponentially with time. Solutions for real cases can be obtained by substituting for the appropriate parameters in Equations (13) to (15).

The Time Lag and The Burst Effect. Though constant-activity reservoir devices give constant release in the steady state, they will initially exhibit release rates higher or lower than the steady-state value, depending on the history of the device. For example, a reservoir device which is loaded with drug and then used immediately will require some time in which to establish the concentration gradient within the membrane. This is called the time lag. Similarly, drug will saturate all the membrane in a device stored for some time before use. When placed in a desorbing solution or put into use, some of the drug in the membrane will desorb at an initially high rate. This is called the burst effect. The magnitude of these two effects is determined by the diffusion coefficient of the drug in the membrane and the membrane thickness. The mathematical development is presented below for the slab.

For a membrane of thickness ℓ, the concentration as a function of time and distance during the approach to the steady state, as given by Crank,[80] is:

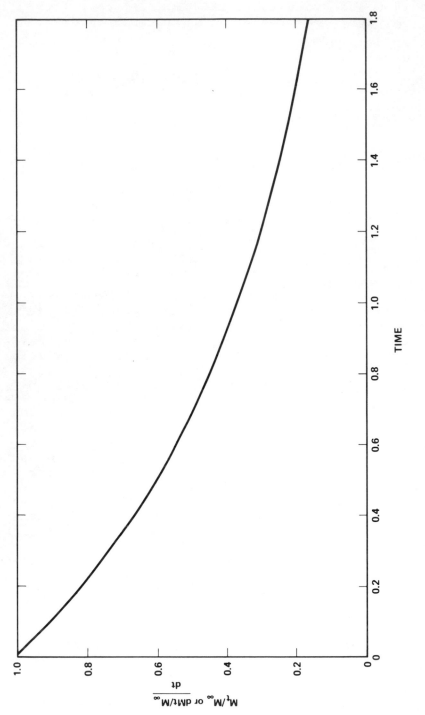

Figure 6.   Fractional release and fractional release rate vs time for a nonconstant activity source diffusing into an infinitely large sink,
showing the exponential decay. (Equations 13 and 14, $ADK/\ell V_1 = 1$).

$$C = C_o + (C_\ell - C_o) \frac{x}{\ell} + \frac{2}{\pi} \sum_{n=1}^{\infty} \frac{C_\ell \cos n\pi - C_o}{n} \sin \frac{n\pi x}{\ell} \exp(-Dn^2\pi^2 t/\ell^2)$$

$$+ \frac{4C_m}{\pi} \sum_{m=0}^{\infty} \frac{1}{2m+1} \sin \frac{(2m+1)\pi x}{\ell} \exp(-D[2m+1]^2\pi^2 t/\ell^2)$$

where C_ℓ is the concentration within the membrane at the outer face $x = \ell$, C_o is the concentration at the inner face $x = 0$, and C_m is the initially uniform concentration in the membrane.

Differentiation of this expression gives the concentration gradient, from which it follows that:

$$J = -D\left(\frac{dC}{dx}\right)_\ell = D\left(\frac{C_o}{\ell} + \frac{2}{\ell} \sum_{n=1}^{\infty} C_o [\cos n\pi] \exp\left[-\frac{D\pi^2 t n^2}{\ell^2}\right]\right.$$

$$\left. - \frac{4C_m}{\ell} \sum_{m=0}^{\infty} \cos([2m+1]\pi) \exp\left[-\frac{D(2m+1)^2\pi^2 t}{\ell^2}\right]\right).$$

We can define the steady-state flux as J_∞, in which case $J_\infty = DC_o/\ell$. In the burst effect case, $C_m = C_o$, and the approximate solution is obtained:

$$\frac{J}{J_\infty} = 1 + 2 \exp\left(\frac{D\pi^2 t}{\ell^2}\right). \tag{16}$$

This is valid for all but short times. Similarly, for the time lag, putting $C_m = 0$, we obtain:

$$\frac{J}{J_\infty} = 1 - 2 \exp\left(-\frac{D\pi^2 t}{\ell^2}\right). \tag{17}$$

The total amount of drug, M_t, which has diffused through a membrane at time t is given by the equation:

$$M_t = \frac{AD(C_o - C_\ell)}{\ell} + \frac{2\ell A}{\pi^2} \sum_{n=1}^{\infty} \frac{C_o \cos n\pi - C_\ell}{n^2} \left(1 - \exp\left[\frac{-Dn^2\pi^2 t}{\ell^2} \right] \right)$$

$$+ \frac{4C_m \ell A}{\pi^2} \sum_{m=0}^{\infty} \frac{1}{(2m+1)^2} \left(1 - \exp\left[\frac{-D[2m+1]^2 \pi^2 t}{\ell^2} \right] \right).$$

For the time lag case, both C_m and C_ℓ are zero and the above equation reduces to:

$$M_t = \frac{ADtC_o}{\ell} - \frac{A\ell C_o}{6} - \frac{A2\ell C_o}{\pi^2} \sum_{n=1}^{\infty} \frac{\cos(n\pi)}{n^2} \exp\left(\frac{-Dn^2\pi^2 t}{\ell^2} \right). \qquad (18)$$

Similarly, for the burst effect case, $C_m = C_o$, $C_\ell = 0$, and

$$M_t = \frac{ADtC_o}{\ell} + \frac{A\ell C_o}{3} - \frac{2\ell C_o A}{\pi^2} \sum_{n=1}^{\infty} \frac{\cos(n\pi)}{n^2} \exp\left(\frac{-Dn^2\pi^2 t}{\ell^2} \right)$$

$$\qquad\qquad (19)$$

$$- \frac{4C_o \ell A}{\pi^2} \sum_{m=0}^{\infty} \frac{1}{(2m+1)^2} \exp\left(\frac{-D[2m+1]^2\pi^2 t}{\ell^2} \right).$$

As $t \to \infty$, the exponential terms in both Equations (18) and (19) vanish. The steady-state results are, for the time lag case, from Equation (18):

$$M_t = \frac{DC_o}{\ell} \left(t - \frac{\ell^2}{6D} \right), \qquad (20)$$

and for the burst effect case from Equation (19):

$$M_t = \frac{DC_o}{\ell} \left(t + \frac{\ell^2}{3D} \right). \qquad (21)$$

If M_t is plotted against time, the intercept, L, of the steady-state portion of the plot on the time axis is given by $-\ell^2/3D$ for the burst effect and $\ell^2/6D$ for the time lag.

Lag time relationships for cylindrical and spherical geometry are given by Crank.[80]

Schematic plots of the results presented in Equations (18)-(21) are presented in Figure 7. In Figure 8 is presented a plot against time of the ratio of the non-steady-state flux to the steady-state flux, J/J_∞. Also indicated on the plot are some multiples of the respective lag times for the two effects. In each case, the release rate is within 1% of the steady-state value after three lag times, L.

It is interesting to note that the time to reach steady state only depends on D and ℓ and not on the amount of drug which must be sorbed or desorbed by a device. The time scale of these devices can be put in perspective by calculating the time lag from Equation (20) for a 100 μ thick membrane in which the drug diffusion coefficient is relatively large, $\underline{i.e.}$, $D \simeq 1 \times 10^{-7}$ cm^2/sec. In this case, the time lag (or burst effect) is only a few minutes. On the other hand, a solution-diffusion membrane of the same thickness and with a diffusion coefficient of the order $10^{-9} - 10^{-10}$ cm^2/sec has a time lag (or burst effect) lasting several hours or even days. Moreover, the extent of this effect increases with the square of the membrane thickness.

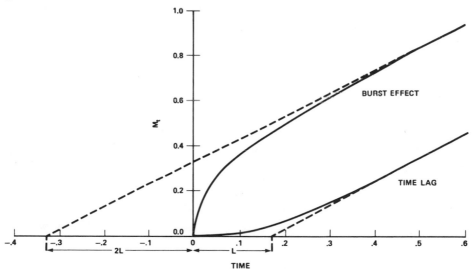

Figure 7. A plot showing the approach to the steady state for a reservoir type device which has been stored for a very long time (the burst effect curve) and for a device which has been freshly made (the time lag curve). ($C_o\ell = 1$, $D/\ell^2 = 1$)

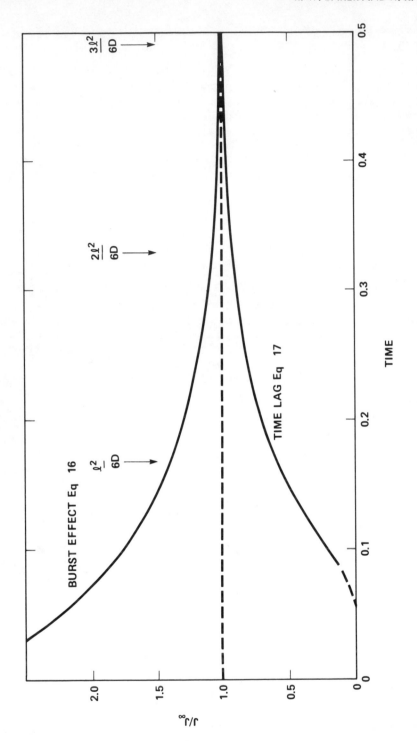

Figure 8. A plot showing the relative release rate curves for a device which has been stored for a very long time (the burst effect curve) and for a device which has been freshly made. $(D/\ell^2 = 1)$.

A good example of the burst-effect phenomenon can be found in data presented by Kincl and Rudel.[84]   Presented in Figure 9 is a plot of their results of release rate of megestrol acetate from cylindrical polydimethylsiloxane capsules of varying length.   The high initial release rate, which persisted for several days, is presumed to be the result of steroid accumulation in the membrane prior to the release rate measurements.

In some cases more complex transient effects are possible, for example, if the drug reservoir is only partially equilibrated with the membrane during storage.   An example of this type of release curve is shown by the data of Shippy, et al.,[85] presented in Figure 9.

Monolithic Devices

In this section, release rate expressions are presented for the case of a drug intimately mixed with the release-rate-controlling membrane in a monolithic device. The drug can be simply dissolved in the monolith or it can be present as a dispersion, and these two cases lead to different release characteristics.   As before, three configurations are of the greatest general importance: the slab, cylinder, and sphere.

Dissolved Drug.   If a homogeneous polymeric film is equilibrated with a drug (for example, by soaking it in a neat liquid or an aqueous solution) drug will dissolve in the polymer and the film can then act as a source for the release of the drug.

We can express desorption of dissolved drug from a slab by either of the series:

$$\frac{M_t}{M_\infty} = 1 - \sum_{n=0}^{\infty} \frac{8 \exp\ (-D[2n+1]^2\pi^2 t/\ell^2)}{(2n+1)^2\pi^2} \tag{22}$$

or

$$\frac{M_t}{M_\infty} = 4\left(\frac{Dt}{\ell^2}\right)^{\frac{1}{2}}\left(\pi^{-\frac{1}{2}} + 2\sum_{n=1}^{\infty}(-1)^n\ \text{ierfc}\ \frac{n\ell}{2\sqrt{Dt}}\right), \tag{23}$$

where M_∞ is the total amount of drug sorbed, M_t is the amount desorbed at time t, and ℓ is the thickness of the device.

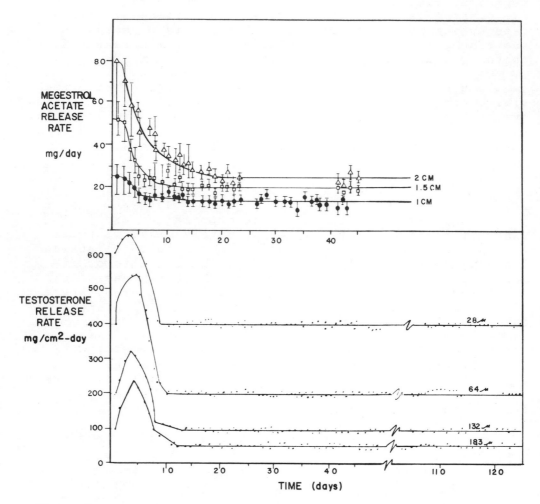

Figure 9.   Burst effect curves for megestrol acetate[84] and
            testosterone[85] from Silastic® cylinders.   In the
            megestrol acetate example, the release rates were
            altered by using capsules of different lengths.   In
            the testosterone example, the release rate was varied
            by altering the membrane thickness.

The above equations are too clumsy for routine use, but fortunately they reduce to two approximations which are valid for different portions of the desorption curve and which are reliable to better than 1%. The early time approximation, which holds over the initial portion of the curve, is derived from Equation (23):

$$\frac{M_t}{M_\infty} = 4 \left(\frac{Dt}{\pi \ell^2} \right)^{\frac{1}{2}} \text{ for } 0 \le \frac{M_t}{M_\infty} \le 0.6 \quad , \tag{24}$$

and the late time approximation, which holds over the final portion of the desorption curve, is derived from Equation (22):

$$\frac{M_t}{M_\infty} = 1 - \frac{8}{\pi^2} \exp \left(\frac{-\pi^2 Dt}{\ell^2} \right) \text{ for } 0.4 \le \frac{M_t}{M_\infty} \le 1.0 \; . \tag{25}$$

Both of these approximations are plotted in Figure 10 which illustrates their different regions of applicability. For simplicity in presenting the results, it has been assumed that $M_\infty = 1$ and $D/\ell^2 = 1$.

In general, the drug release rate at any time is of more interest than the accumulated total drug release. This is easily obtained by differentiating equations (24) and (25) which give:

$$\frac{dM_t}{dt} = 2M_\infty \left(\frac{D}{\pi \ell^2 t} \right)^{\frac{1}{2}} \tag{26}$$

for the early time approximation, and

$$\frac{dM_t}{dt} = \frac{8DM_\infty}{\ell^2} \exp \left(- \frac{\pi^2 Dt}{\ell^2} \right) \tag{27}$$

for the late time approximation.

Figure 11 shows a plot of these two approximations against time. Again, for simplicity, M_∞ and D/ℓ^2 have been set equal to unity. The release rate falls off as $t^{-\frac{1}{2}}$ over the first 60% of the release after which it decays in an exponential manner following Equation (27).

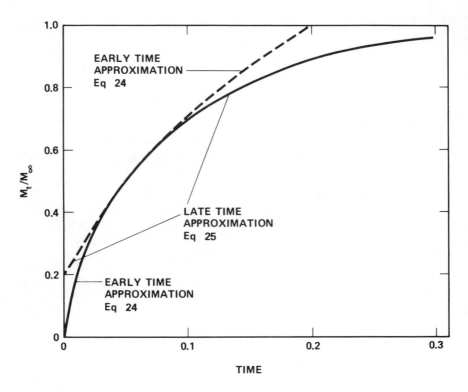

Figure 10.   Plots of the fraction of drug desorbed from
a slab as a function of time using the early
time and late time approximations. The full
line shows the portion of the curve over
which the approximations are valid.
$(D/\ell^2 = 1)$.

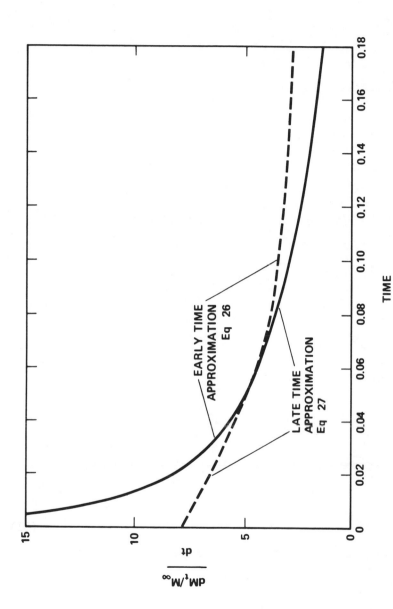

Figure 11.   Plots of the release rate of drug initially dissolved in a slab as a function of time, using the early time and late time approximations. The full line shows the portion of the curve over which the approximations are valid. $(D/\ell^2 = 1)$.

The time required to release half of the total dissolved drug ($t_{\frac{1}{2}}$) and the release rate at this time are often useful in quick feasibility calculations. From Equations (22) and (23) we can show that:

$$t_{\frac{1}{2}} = 0.0492 \, \frac{\ell^2}{D} \, , \qquad (28)$$

and from (24) and (26) we can write the release rate at the half time as:

$$\left(\frac{dM_t}{dt}\right)_{t_{\frac{1}{2}}} = \frac{16DM_{\infty}}{\pi \ell^2} \qquad (29)$$

Figure 12 shows an experimental desorption curve obtained with a Hydron® contact lens previously soaked in an aqueous 4% pilocarpine nitrate solution. The solid line has been calculated from Equations (24) and (25) assuming $\ell^2/D = 3700$ sec. The agreement between the calculated line and experiment is good even though the contact lens was not a perfectly flat disc.

Mathematical solutions for desorption of solutes from devices of other geometries can be found in standard sources.[80,81] As in the case of the slab, these solutions are given in terms of an early time and a late time approximation. For the cylinder, the early time approximation for the fractional release is given by:

$$\frac{M_t}{M_{\infty}} = 4\left(\frac{Dt}{r\pi^2}\right)^{\frac{1}{2}} - \frac{Dt}{r^2} \qquad (30)$$

which is accurate for $M_t/M_{\infty} \leqslant 0.4$. The release rate is given by:

$$\frac{dM_t/M_{\infty}}{dt} = 2\left(\frac{D}{r^2\pi t}\right)^{\frac{1}{2}} - \frac{D}{r^2} \, . \qquad (31)$$

The late time approximations are:

$$\frac{M_t}{M_{\infty}} = 1 - \frac{4}{(2.405)^2} \exp\left[-\frac{(2.405)^2 \, Dt}{r^2}\right] \qquad (32)$$

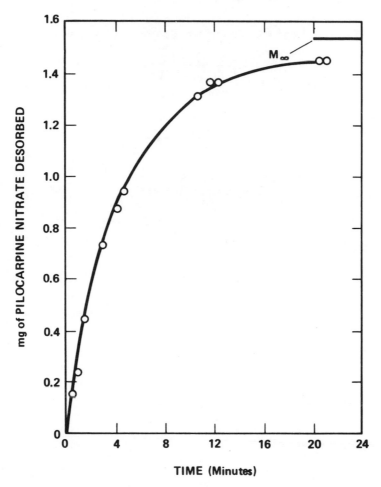

Figure 12. Rate of desorption of pilocarpine nitrate from a 70 mg Hydron® contact lens previously equilibrated with an aqueous solution of 4% pilocarpine nitrate.

which is accurate for $M_t/M_\infty > 0.6$, and

$$\frac{dM_t/M_\infty}{dt} = \frac{4D}{r^2} \exp\left[\frac{-(2.405)^2 \, Dt}{r^2}\right].$$

(33)

For the sphere, the early time approximations are:

$$\frac{M_t}{M_\infty} = 6\left(\frac{Dt}{r^2\pi}\right)^{1/2} - \frac{3Dt}{r^2}$$

(34)

which is valid for $M_t/M_\infty < 0.4$, and

$$\frac{dM_t/M_\infty}{dt} = 3\left(\frac{D}{r^2\pi t}\right)^{1/2} - \frac{3D}{r^2}.$$

(35)

The late time solutions are:

$$\frac{M_t}{M_\infty} = 1 - \frac{6}{\pi^2} \exp\left(\frac{-\pi^2 Dt}{r^2}\right)$$

(36)

which is valid for $M_t/M_\infty > 0.6$, and

$$\frac{dM_t/M_\infty}{dt} = \frac{6Dt}{r^2} \exp\left(\frac{-\pi^2 Dt}{r^2}\right).$$

(37)

The complete curves for fractional release and release rate for the slab, cylinder, and sphere are
presented in Figure 13. These have been normalized by
assuming $D/\ell^2 = 1$ for the slab and $D/r^2 = 1$ for the
cylinder and sphere.

Dispersed Drug. If the drug is dispersed as a solid
in the membrane phase instead of being dissolved, the
release kinetics are altered. In this case, when the
total concentration of drug, C_0, (dissolved plus dispersed) is larger than the solubility in the membrane,
C_s, the release kinetics have been derived by T. Higuchi[86]
using the model illustrated.

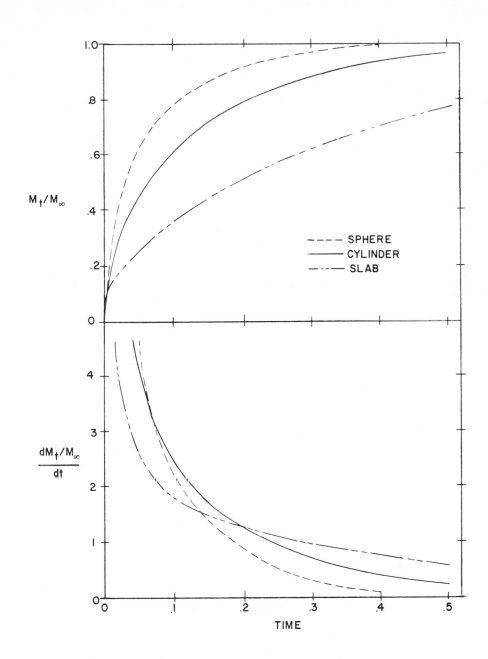

Figure 13.   Fractional release and release rate vs time
             for drug dissolved in a slab, cylinder, and
             sphere. $(d/\ell^2$ or $D/r^2 = 1)$.

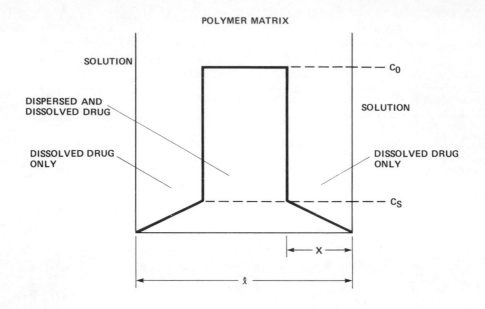

In this model, it is assumed that solid drug dissolves from the surface layer of the device first and when this layer becomes exhausted of drug the next layer begins to be depleted. The interface between the region containing only dissolved drug thus moves into the interior as a front. The validity of the Higuchi model has been experimentally demonstrated numerous times. In addition, the movement of the dissolving drug front was actually monitored under the microscope by Roseman and W. Higuchi.[87]

The proof of T. Higuchi is straightforward and is given below for completeness. Starting from Fick's law for the slab we can write:

$$\frac{dM_t}{dt} = \frac{ADC_s}{x} ,$$

and at time t, from mass balance considerations,

$$\frac{2x}{\ell} = \frac{M_t + AxC_s/2}{M_\infty} .$$

Combining the above equations,

$$\frac{dM_t}{dt} = \frac{ADC_s M_\infty}{M_t} \left(\frac{2}{\ell} - \frac{AC_s}{2M_\infty} \right).$$

Integrating gives

$$M_t^2 = ADC_s \left(\frac{2}{\ell} - \frac{AC_s}{2M_\infty} \right) M_\infty t ,$$

and substituting

$$M_\infty = \frac{AC_o \ell}{2}$$

and rearranging gives

$$M_t = A \left[DtC_s (2C_o - C_s) \right]^{\frac{1}{2}} \tag{38}$$

$$\simeq A(2DtC_s C_o)^{\frac{1}{2}} \text{ for } C_o \gg C_s . \tag{39}$$

The release rate at any time is then given by:

$$\frac{dM_t}{dt} = \frac{A}{2} \left[\frac{DC_s}{t} (2C_o - C_s) \right]^{\frac{1}{2}} \tag{40}$$

$$\simeq \frac{A}{2} \left[\frac{2DC_s C_o}{t} \right]^{\frac{1}{2}} \text{ for } C_o \gg C_s . \tag{41}$$

The point of exhaustion (or the time when the last solid drug just dissolves, t_∞) can be calculated from (39) as:

$$t_\infty = \frac{\ell^2 C_o}{8DC_s} . \tag{42}$$

These equations have almost the same form as the initial
release of dissolved drug given by Equation (24) and (26)
but, instead of tailing off at late times, the $t^{-\frac{1}{2}}$ relationship holds over almost the complete release curve,
i.e., until the drug concentration in the center of the
membrane falls below the saturation value. Figure 14
shows a plot of Equation (41) for different drug loadings
in the same matrix. For simplicity of presentation, it
has been assumed that $\ell^2/8D = 1$ and $AC_S\ell/2 = 1$. The
simplifying assumption that $C_O \gg C_S$ is reasonable for
almost all polymer-drug dispersions containing more than
∿5 wt% drug and is often valid for polymer-drug dispersions containing as little as 1 wt% drug.

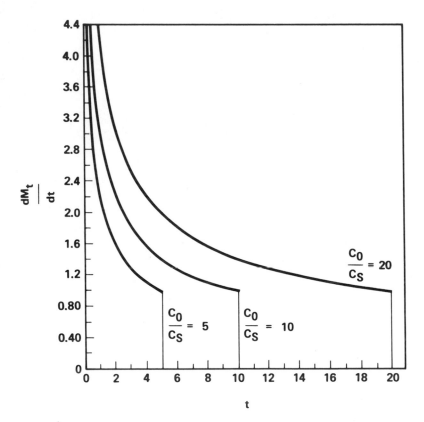

Figure 14.   Plots showing the release rate of drug from
              a slab containing different loadings of dis-
              persed solid drug. ($\ell^2/8D = 1$ $AC_S\ell/2 = 1$)

From Equation (40) it follows that the release rate is proportional to the square root of the drug loading and can thus be easily varied by incorporating more or less drug. Furthermore, although the release rate pattern is by no means constant, it is considerably less variable than the dissolved drug case.

An example of the release rate of a drug from a silicone elastomer slab containing dispersed drug is presented in Figure 15. The data are taken from Haleblian, et al.[69] The amount of drug released is seen to increase with the square root of time and approximately with the square root of the loading, in accordance with Equation (39). Numerous other examples of this type of behavior can be found in the publications of Simonelli, W. Higuchi, et al.,[88-93] and Sjögren, et al.[94-96]

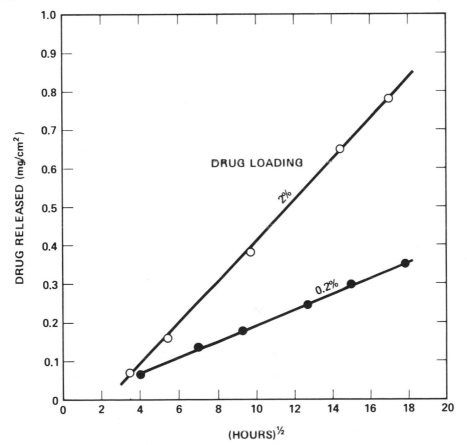

Figure 15.   Release of micronized chlormadinone acetate from silicone elastomer into water vs the square root of time.[69]

The solution for the release kinetics for cylindrical geometry when $C_o \gg C_s$, has been given previously by Roseman and W. Higuchi.[87,97] In this case, the expressions do not reduce to a simple form as in the case of the slab. Thus, the drug release rate at time t is:

$$\frac{dM_t}{dt} = \frac{2\pi C_s D \ell}{\ln[M_\infty/(M_\infty - M_t)]^{\frac{1}{2}}} \, , \tag{43}$$

or in dimensionless terms:

$$\frac{dM_t/M_\infty}{dt} = \frac{-4C_s D}{r_o^2 C_o \ln(1 - M_t/M_\infty)} \tag{44}$$

Rearranging the above equation gives the expression for the fractional drug loss at any time t:

$$\left(1 - \frac{M_t}{M_\infty}\right)\left(\ln\left[1 - \frac{M_t}{M_\infty}\right]\right) + \frac{M_t}{M_\infty} = \frac{4C_s D}{C_o r_o^2} \cdot t \tag{45}$$

From (45) we can obtain a dimensionless plot of M_t/M_∞ vs t.

In principle, it is possible to substitute for M_t/M_∞ into Equation (44) and obtain the drug release rate as a function of time, but it is more practical to compute the differential of Equation (45) using the digital computer.

From Equation (45), the device becomes exhausted when $M_t = M_\infty$, in which case

$$t_\infty = \frac{C_o r_o^2}{4DC_s} \, . \tag{46}$$

Comparing Equations (44), (45), and (46) for the cylinder with their equivalent equations for the slab, namely:

$$\frac{dM_t/M_\infty}{dt} = \frac{4C_s D}{\ell^2 C_o} \frac{1}{M_t/M_\infty} \, ,$$

$$\left(\frac{M_t}{M_\infty}\right)^2 = \frac{8C_s D}{C_o \ell^2} \cdot t \, ,$$

and

$$t_\infty = \frac{\ell^2 C_o}{8DC_s}$$

shows a remarkable similarity in that both sets are functions of the square of their linear dimensions and have the same dependence on the term DC_s/C_o. The cylinder, however, shows a more marked decay in release rate as time progresses.

An example of the release of a dispersed drug from a cylindrical Silastic® device is given in the work of Cornette and Duncan,[98] which is reproduced in Figure 16. The release rate falls off approximately according to the $t^{-\frac{1}{2}}$ law. The initial drug loading, in micrograms per centimeter of length of the cylinder, is shown on the graph. The dependence of release rate at a given time on initial loading is complex, as shown by Equation (45). Several additional examples are presented by Roseman and W. Higuchi[87,97] and elsewhere.[99,100] A point worth noting here is that for dissolved drug, the fraction released at a given time is independent of initial loading, whereas for dispersed drug, the fractional release at a given time decreases with increasing loading, and the relationship between release rate and loading depends on the geometry of the device. For both types of device, however, the release falls off according to a $t^{-\frac{1}{2}}$ law for approximately the first 50% of the drug. The solution for spherical geometry is similar to the slab and cylinder and it can be shown that the drug release rate is given by the expression:

$$\frac{dM_t/M_\infty}{dt} = \frac{3C_s D}{r_o^2 C_o} \left(\frac{[1-M_t/M_\infty]^{1/3}}{1 - [1-M_t/M_\infty]^{1/3}} \right), \tag{47}$$

which on integration gives:

$$\frac{3}{2}\left(1 - \left[1 - \frac{M_t}{M_\infty}\right]^{2/3}\right) - \frac{M_t}{M_\infty} = \frac{3DC_s}{r_o^2 C_o} \cdot t . \tag{48}$$

From this it follows that the device becomes exhausted of solid drug at a time, t_∞, given by:

$$t_\infty = \frac{r_o^2 C_o}{6DC_s} . \tag{49}$$

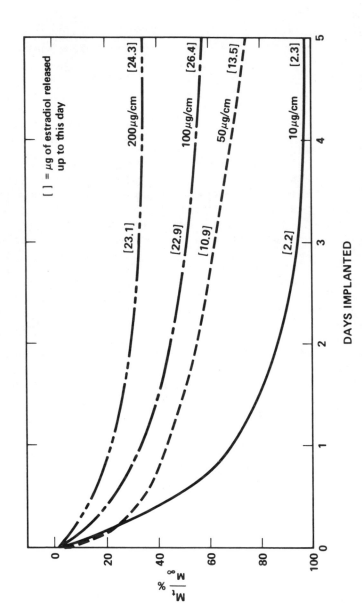

Figure 16.   In vivo release of ^{3}H – estradiol from Silastic® implants with varying concentrations of dispersed steroid.[98]

As with the slab, it is not possible to express the release rate as a single function of time.

A similar result for the release rate from a spherical
dispersion has been given previously by T. Higuchi.[101]
Some examples of drug release from spherical dispersions
are described by T. Higuchi and by Luzzi, et al.[102]

A comparison of release kinetics for the three important geometries is presented in Figure 17. The curves
have been normalized so that all the drug is released at
$t_\infty = 1$, i.e., the area under all three curves is identical. It was assumed in all cases that $C_O >> C_S$. The three
curves are initially similar, the most important differences showing up close to the point of drug depletion.

If the drug loading is not greatly in excess of the
drug solubility, a complex situation arises, the kinetics
of which involve a fusion of the dissolved and dispersed
cases. An example of such a situation can be found in
the work of Lapidus and Lordi.[103,104] Another special
case, the codelivery of two noninteracting drugs, has
been treated by Singh and co-workers.[105]

Boundary Layer Effects

We have assumed to this point that drug release is
solely determined by the rate of diffusion of drug to
the surface of the device. It was assumed that this surface is maintained at zero concentration essentially
throughout the life of the device. This situation is
sometimes not attained in practice because of the slow
transport of the drug away from the membrane surface.
The concentration of drug at the membrane surface is then
finite, and under some circumstances can reach appreciable
values. In the extreme case, the drug concentration in
the fluid immediately surrounding the device, the so-
called boundary layer or unstirred layer, can reach the
drug's solubility, C_S, at which point the device would
cease delivering drug. Boundary-layer effects are most
serious with relatively water-insoluble drugs. With
these, the driving force for diffusion in the boundary
layer is low and the drug concentration can rapidly
approach saturation at the surface of the device.

The boundary-layer problem in vivo is hard to quantify
because the hydrodynamic conditions are usually unknown.
However, we can be sure that the stirring in many body
cavities is poor and one approach to the boundary layer

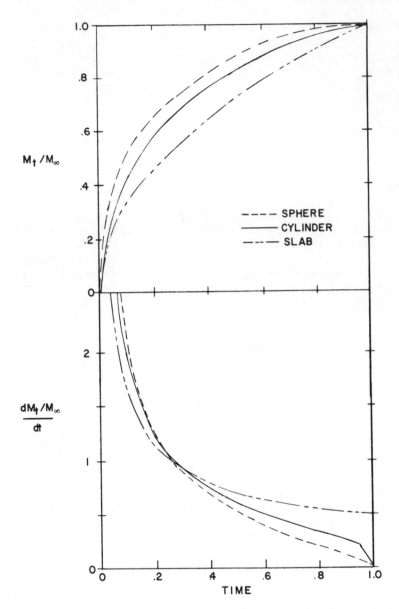

Figure 17.   Theoretical fractional release and release rate <u>vs</u>. time for a dispersed drug in a slab, cylinder, and sphere.

problem is to assume that the fluid surrounding a device is completely stagnant. In this case the rate of build-up of the drug in the stagnant fluid is given by Crank[80] as:

$$\frac{C_x}{C_s} = \text{erfc} \ \frac{x}{2\sqrt{Dt}} - \exp \ (\gamma x + \gamma^2 Dt) \ \text{erfc} \left(\frac{x}{2\sqrt{Dt}} + \gamma\sqrt{Dt} \right).$$

In this equation, x is the distance from the surface into the surrounding medium and γ is a parameter defined for our case as $\gamma = J/C_s D$, where J is the flux of drug away from the surface of the device. Figure 18 is a graphical solution to the above equation taken from Crank. In this figure, the relative concentration in the surrounding medium, C/C_s, is plotted against the dimensionless distance parameter $x/(4Dt)^{\frac{1}{2}}$ for several values of the dimensionless flux away from the surface of the device, $\gamma(Dt^{\frac{1}{2}})$. As this flux increases, the drug concentration approaches the solubility at progressively smaller distances from the surface. (The same qualitative conclusion will hold, of course, in stirred as well as unstirred systems.) To put the results of Figure 18 into usable form, we will make the assumption that $D = 2 \times 10^{-6} \ \text{cm}^2/\text{sec}$, a reasonable value for drugs in aqueous media at body temperature. If we also arbitrarily assume that J in $\mu\text{g/cm}^2\text{-hr}$ is numerically identical to C_s in $\mu\text{g/cm}^3$, then $\gamma = 139 \ \text{cm}^{-1}$. With this value, we can calculate $\gamma(Dt)^{\frac{1}{2}}$ and $(4Dt)^{\frac{1}{2}}$ and thus the concentration profiles in the surrounding medium.

The result of this calculation is presented in Figure 19. The results are presented as relative concentration vs distance for various times, showing the rate at which the external concentration approaches the saturation value in an unstirred medium. The effect of this concentration buildup on the release rate can now be calculated. If we define the flux into a well mixed solution maintained at zero concentration of drug as J_{max}, then flux at any time, J_t, in the case of an unstirred solution is given by:

$$J_t = J_{max} \left(1 - \left[\frac{C}{C_s} \right]_{x=0} \right). \tag{50}$$

Such a plot, for our assumed values of D and γ, is presented in Figure 20.

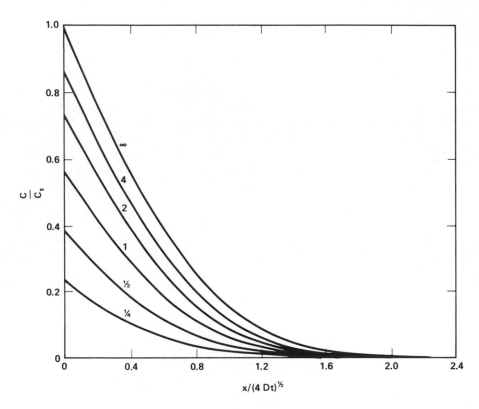

Figure 18. Concentration distribution for diffusion
            from a surface into a semi-infinite medium.
            Numbers on curves are values of $\gamma(Dt)^{\frac{1}{2}}$.

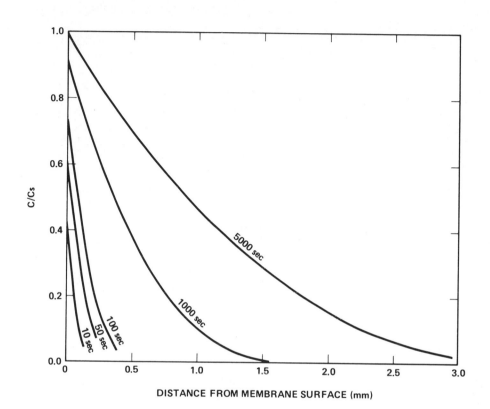

Figure 19.   This figure shows the buildup in drug con-
             centration near the surface of a membrane
             releasing drug into an unstirred fluid at
             different times.   In this example, we have
             assumed a drug diffusion coefficient of
             2×10^{-6} cm^2/sec and a ratio of J_{max}
             (μg/cm^2-hr) to C_s (ppm) of 1.

Obviously, the results in Figure 19 are tied to the
assumption that the flux, J_{max}, is identical to the solubility in $\mu g/cm^3$, an arbitrary but not unreasonable
assumption. However these results are easily scaled for
other values of J_{max}/C_s and the effect of the build up
in concentration on the flux is shown in Figure 20. For
real cases, where the release rate into a well-stirred
medium and the drug solubility and diffusivity are known,
the procedure used above can be reproduced to calculate
the actual effect on release rate in an unstirred system.

Of course, even in the body limited stirring does
exist and another approach to calculating the boundary-
layer effect is to assume a stagnant layer of arbitrary
thickness around the device. The reduction in flux due
to the build up in concentration in solution at the membrane surface is again given by Equation (50). The diffusion of drug through the boundary layer is given by
Fick's law:

$$J = \frac{DC_{x=0}}{\lambda} , \qquad (51)$$

where γ is the boundary-layer thickness, and $C_{x=0}$ is the
concentration of drug immediately adjacent to the membrane surface. It is assumed that the drug concentration
outside the boundary layer is zero. Combining Equations
(50) and (51):

$$\frac{J}{J_{max}} = \frac{1}{1 + \frac{J_{max}\lambda}{C_s D}} . \qquad (52)$$

Figure 21 shows a plot of J/J_{max} vs the ratio J_{max}/C_s
for various boundary-layer thicknesses, assuming a diffusion coefficient, D, in water of 2×10^{-6} cm^2/sec.
Boundary layers in stirred systems are typically of the
order 100 μ but in the body they can be much larger.

Both approaches to this problem show that the parameter which determines the extent of the boundary-layer
problem is the quotient J_{max}/C_s.

It would appear that many of the experimental studies
of controlled-release medication were influenced by
boundary-layer effects. The frequently poor agreement
between in vitro and in vivo release rates with insoluble drugs and very high release rate devices can

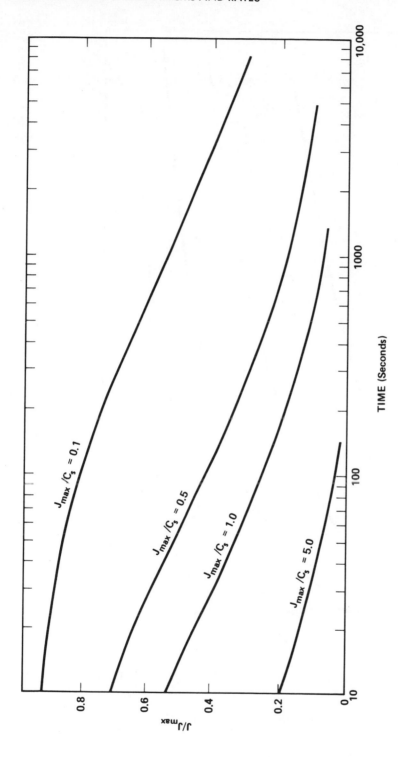

Figure 20. The rate of drop in flux from the maximum value, J_{max}, for different ratios of J_{max}/C_s in a stagnant fluid, where J_{max} is in $\mu g/cm^2$-hr and C_s is in ppm.

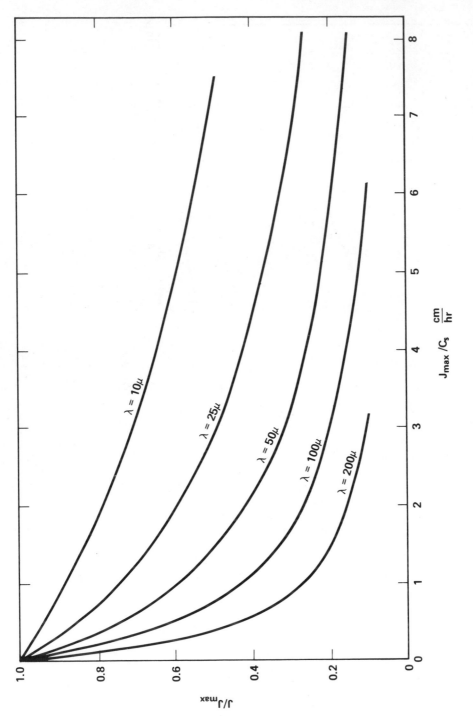

Figure 21.   A plot of the fractional decrease in drug release rate against J_{max}/C_s with boundary layers of increasing thickness.

commonly be attributed to this phenomenon - even in some
of those cases, for example, where the disparity is
attributed to the encapsulation of an implanted device
by fibrous tissue. In some studies of reservoir-type
devices, it has been noted that the release rate in
vivo was independent of the membrane thickness, but increased with membrane area, a result consistent with a
boundary-layer effect.[106-109] In the design of drug
delivery systems the quotient J_{max}/C_s should be maintained at as low a value as possible to avoid these
effects.

In closing, it might be noted that many drugs, particularly steroids, are quite hydrophobic and they
partition very effectively into polymeric materials.
In many cases of potential interest, therefore, the permeability of the membrane may be comparable to or even
greater than that of water.

V.   CONCLUSIONS

The past few years have seen a rapid development in
the field of controlled-release systems, particularly
as applied to pharmaceuticals. At the present time,
this field is particularly fertile, with a number of
important applications emerging from the laboratory. We
have tried to show here in detail how membrane-moderated
devices and the simple application of diffusion laws can
lead to controlled release of drugs (or other agents)
according to zero-order or first-order kinetics or more
complex patterns.

Because of its favorable biocompatibility, silicone
rubber emerged as the most important material in this
new field, but other materials are under investigation
in those applications where compatibility demands are
less stringent. Some of these newer materials offer
specific advantages such as mechanical properties, ease
of fabrication, or release characteristics. The release-
rate relationships presented here are generally applicable for diffusion-controlled devices, regardless of
their constitutive elements. These relationships may be
summarized as follows: For reservoir devices, release
rate can be zero-order providing the device is designed
to maintain unit thermodynamic activity immediately inside the rate-limiting membrane. For monolithic devices
with dissolved drug, release rate falls according to a
$t^{-\frac{1}{2}}$ law for about the first half of the device life, and

then it falls exponentially. For monolithic devices with
a large amount of excess dispersed drug, release rate
falls according to the $t^{-\frac{1}{2}}$ law essentially throughout
life. However refined these controlled-release devices
become, they are still subject to the influence of
boundary-layer effects in use, and care must be exercised
both in the initial design and in interpreting results.

    As noted, this field is in a state of rapid ferment,
and we can expect the development and application of
progressively more sophisticated and effective devices
based on elementary principles.

ACKNOWLEDGMENTS

    The authors are indebted to several members of the
ALZA staff: R. M. Gale and D. Hernandez for assistance
in the measurements shown in Figures 4 and 12, J. Scott
Hamilton for the computer programming that resulted in
Figure 17, and J. Bashaw, A. S. Michaels, and F. Theeuwes
for a number of useful discussions.

REFERENCES

1. O. R. Lunt, J. Agr. Food Chem., 19 797 (1971).

2. G. G. Allan, C. S. Chopra, J. F. Friedhoff,
    R. I. Gara, M. W. Maggi, A. N. Neogi, S. C. Roberts,
    and R. M. Wilkins, Chem. Tech., March 1973.

3. J. V. Swintosky, Indian J. Pharm., 25, 360 (1963).

4. G. Nairn, Can. Pharm. J., 102, 336 (1969).

5. A. Williams, Sustained Release Pharmaceuticals,
    Noyes Development Corporation, Park Ridge, N. J.
    (1969).

6. J. Folkman and D. M. Long, Jr., J. Surg. Res., 4,
    139 (1964).

7. J. Folkman and V. H. Mark, Trans. N. Y. Acad. Sci.,
    Ser. II, 30, 1187 (1968).

8. J. Folkman, S. Winsey, and T. Moghul, Anesthesiology,
    29, 410 (1968).

9. J. Folkman, V. H. Mark, F. Ervin, K. Suematsu, and
    R. Hagiwara,, Anesthesiology, 29, 419 (1968).

10. K. G. Powers, J. Parasitology, 51, Sec 2, 53 (1965).

11. P. Bass, R. A. Purdon, and J. N. Wiley, Nature, 208,
    591 (1965).

12. J. Dziuk and B. Cook, Endocrinology, 78, 208 (1966).

13. F. A. Kincl, G. Benagiano, and I. Angee, Steroids,
    11, 673 (1968).

14. K. Sundaram and F. A. Kincl, Steroids, 12, 517
    (1968).

15. P. Kratochvil, G. Benagiano, and F. A. Kincl,
    Steroids, 15, 505 (1970).

16. S. Friedman, S. S. Koide, and F. A. Kincl, Steroids,
    15, 679 (1970).

17. F. A. Kincl, K. Sundaram, C. C. Chang, and
    H. W. Rudel, Acta Endocrinologica, 64, 253 (1970).

18. F. A. Kincl, I. Angee, C. C. Chang, and H. W. Rudel,
    Acta Endocrinologica, 64, 508 (1970).

19. H. Croxatto, S. Diaz, R. Vera, M. Etchart, and
    P. Atria, _Am. J. Obst. and Gynec._, 105, 1135 (1969).

20. H. J. Tatum, E. M. Coutinho, J. A. Filho, and
    A. R. S. Sant'anna, _Am. J. Obst. and Gynec._, 105,
    1139 (1969).

21. D. R. Mishell, M. Talas, A. F. Parlow, and D. L.
    Moyer, _Contraception_, 107, 100 (1970).

22. D. R. Mishell and M. E. Lumkin, _Fertility and
    Sterility_, 21, 99 (1970).

23. A. Scommegna, G. N. Pandya, M. Christ, A. W. Lee,
    and M. R. Cohen, _Fertility and Sterility_, 21, 201
    (1970).

24. A. S. Lifchez and A. Scommegna, _Fertility and
    Sterility_, 21, 426 (1970).

25. H. J. Tatum, _Contraception_, 1, 253 (1970).

26. M. C. Chang, J. H. Casas, and D. M. Hunt, _Nature_,
    226, 1262 (1970).

27. M. R. N. Prasad, S. P. Singh, and M. Rajalakshmi,
    Contraception, 2, 165 (1970).

28. E. M. Coutinho, D. A. M. Ferreira, H. Prates, and
    F. Kincl, _J. Reprod. Fert._, 23, 345 (1970).

29. E. M. Coutinho, C. E. R. Mattos, A. R. S. Sant'anna,
    J. A. Filho, M. C. Silva, and H. J. Tatum, _Contra-
    ception_, 2, 313 (1970).

30. H. H. Horne, Jr., J. M. Scott, and R. H. Underwood,
    International J. Fertility, 15, 210 (1970).

31. J. Hubacek, K. Kliment, J. Dusek, and J. Hubacek,
    J. Biomed. Mater. Res., 1, 387 (1967).

32. D. F. Williams, _Bio-medical Engineering_, April 1971,
    p. 152.

33. J. Autian, _Ann. N. Y. Acad. Sci._, 146, 251 (1968).

34.   R. Lefaux, Practical Toxicology of Plastics, Iliffe
      Books, Ltd., London, 1968.

35.   D. D. Stromberg and C. A. Wiederhielm, Amer. J.
      Physiol., 219, 928 (1970).

36.   E. W. Merrill, U. S. Patent #3,608,549 (Sept. 28,
      1971).

37.   P. Siegel and J. R. Atkinson, J. Appl. Physiol.,
      30, 900 (1971).

38.   J. M. R. Delgado, F. V. DeFeudis, R. H. Roth,
      D. K. Ryugo, and B. M. Mitruka, Arch. Int.
      Pharmacodynamie Thérapie, 198, 9 (1972).

39.   J. W. Miles, G. W. Pearce, and J. E. Woehst, Agri-
      cultural and Food Chem., 10, 240 (1962).

40.   J. T. Whitlaw, Jr., and E. S. Evans, Jr., J. Economic
      Entomology, 61, 889 (1968).

41.   J. L. Bach, Modern Hospital, June 1970.

42.   H. B. Hopfenberg and J. J. Tulis, Modern Plastics,
      July 1970, p. 110.

43.   A. S. Michaels and H. J. Bixler in Progress in
      Separation and Purification, Vol. I, E. S. Perry
      (Ed.), Interscience, New York, 1968, p. 143-186.

44.   W. R. Lieb and W. D. Stein, Nature, 224, 240 (1969).

45.   W. D. Stein and S. Nir, J. Membrane Biol., 5, 246
      (1971).

46.   W. R. Lieb and W. D. Stein, Nature New Biology, 234,
      220 (1971).

47.   J. Crank and G. S. Park (Eds.), Diffusion in Poly-
      mers, Academic Press, London, 1968.

48.   C. E. Rogers in Physics and Chemistry of the Organic
      Solid State, D. Fox, M. M. Labes, and A. Weissberger
      (Eds.), Interscience Publishers, New York, 1965,
      pp. 509-635.

49.   F. Grün, Experimentia, 3, 490 (1947). Reproduced
      in English in Rubber Chem. and Tech., 22, 316 (1949).

50. G. S. Park, _Trans. Far. Soc._, **46**, 684 (1950).

51. G. S. Park, _Trans. Far. Soc._, **47**, 1007 (1951).

52. V. Stannett, Chap. 2, in _Diffusion in Polymers_, J. Crank and G. S. Park (Eds.), Academic Press, London (1968).

53. C. M. Hansen, _J. Paint Tech._, **39**, 104 (1967).

54. C. M. Hansen, _J. Paint Tech._, **39**, 505 (1967).

55. C. M. Hansen, _Ind. Eng. Chem. Prod. Res. Devel._, **8**, 2 (1969).

56. H. Burrell, _Official Digest_, Oct. 1955, p. 726.

57. H. Burrell, _Official Digest_, Nov. 1957, p. 1159.

58. H. Burrell, _J. Paint Tech._, **40**, 197 (1968).

59. E. P. Lieberman, _Official Digest_, Jan. 1962, p. 30.

60. R. F. Blanks and J. M. Prausnitz, _Ind. Eng. Chem. Fundamentals_, **3**, 1 (1964).

61. J. D. Crowley, G. S. Teague, Jr., and J. W. Lowe, Jr., _J. Paint Tech._, **38**, 269 (1966).

62. J. D. Crowley, G. S. Teague, Jr., and J. W. Lowe, Jr., _J. Paint Tech._, **39**, 19 (1967).

63. J. P. Teas, _J. Paint Tech._, **40**, 19 (1968).

64. J. G. Helpinstill and M. Van Winkle, _Ind. Eng. Chem. Proc. Des. Devel._, **7**, 213 (1968).

65. A. Beerbower and T. R. Dickey, _Amer. Soc. Lubrication Eng. Trans._, **12**, 1 (1969).

66. K. L. Hoy, _J. Paint Tech._, **42**, 76 (1970).

67. L. A. Utracki, _J. Appl. Poly. Sci._, **16**, 1167 (1972).

68. H. Burrell and B. Immergut in _Polymer Handbook_, J. Brandrup and E. H. Immergut (Eds.), Interscience, New York, 1967.

69. J. Haleblian, R. Runkel, N. Mueller, J. Cristopherson, and K. Ng, _J. Pharm. Sci._, **60**, 541 (1971).

70. G. L. Flynn and T. J. Roseman, J. Pharm. Sci., 60, 1788 (1971).

71. C. F. Most, J. App. Poly. Sci., 14, 1019 (1970).

72. E. R. Garrett and P. B. Chemburkar, J. Pharm. Sci., 57, 949 (1968).

73. Ibid, p. 1401.

74. M. Nakano and N. K. Patel, J. Pharm. Sci., 59, 77 (1970).

75. S. Prager and F. A. Long, J. Amer. Chem. Soc., 73, 4072 (1951).

76. R. J. Kokes, F. A. Long, and J. L. Hoard, J. Phys. Chem., 20, 1711 (1952).

77. F. A. Long and R. J. Kokes, J. Amer. Chem. Soc., 75, 2232 (1953).

78. G. S. Park, Trans. Far. Soc., 46, 684 (1950).

79. G. Blyholder and S. Prager, J. Phys. Chem., 64, 702 (1960).

80. J. Crank, The Mathematics of Diffusion, Oxford University Press, London (1956).

81. H. S. Carslaw and J. C. Jaeger, Conduction of Heat in Solids, Oxford University Press, London (1959).

82. R. W. Baker, ALZA Corp., unpublished results.

83. B. H. Vickery, G. I. Erickson, J. P. Bennett, N. S. Mueller, and J. K. Haleblian, Biology of Reproduction, 3, 154 (1970).

84. F. A. Kincl and H. W. Rudel, Acta Endocrinologica Supplementum, p. 5 (1970).

85. R. L. Shippy, S. T. Hwang, R. G. Bunge, J. Biomed. Mater. Res., 7, 95 (1973).

86. T. Higuchi, J. Pharm. Sci., 50, 874 (1961).

87. T. J. Roseman and W. I. Higuchi, J. Pharm. Sci., 59, 353 (1970).

88.   S. J. Desai, A. P. Simonelli, and W. I. Higuchi,
      J. Pharm. Sci., 54, 1459 (1965).

89.   S. J. Desai, P. Singh, A. P. Simonelli, and W. I.
      Higuchi, J. Pharm. Sci., 55, 1224 (1966).

90.   Ibid., p. 1230.

91.   Ibid., p. 1235.

92.   J. B. Schwartz, A. P. Simonelli, and W. I. Higuchi,
      J. Pharm. Sci., 57, 274 (1968).

93.   Ibid., p. 278.

94.   J. Sjögren and L. Fryklöf, Särtryck ur Farmacetisk
      Revy, 59, 171 (1960).

95.   J. Sjögren, Acta Pharmaceutica Suecica, 8, 153
      (1971).

96.   P. F. D'Arcy, J. P. Griffin, J. S. Jenkins, W. F.
      Kirk, and A. W. C. Peacock, J. Pharm. Sci., 60,
      1028 (1971).

97.   T. J. Roseman, J. Pharm. Sci., 61, 46 (1972).

98.   J. C. Cornette and G. W. Duncan, Contraception, 1,
      339 (1970).

99.   B. B. Pharriss and J. W. Hendix, Advances in Planned
      Parenthood, Vol. V., Excerpta Medica Foundation,
      Amsterdam, 1970, p. 149-150.

100. D. R. Kalkwarf, M. R. Sikov, L. Smith, and R. Gordon,
      Contraception, 6, 423 (1972).

101. T. Higuchi, J. Pharm. Sci., 52, 1145 (1963).

102. L. A. Luzzi, M. A. Zoglio, H. V. Maulding, J. Pharm.
      Sci., 59, 338 (1970).

103. H. Lapidus and N. G. Lordi, J. Pharm. Sci., 55, 840
      (1966).

104. H. Lapidus and N. G. Lordi, J. Pharm. Sci., 57,
      1292 (1968).

105. P. Singh, S. J. Desai, A. P. Simonelli, and W. I. Higuchi, J. Pharm. Sci., 56, 1542 (1967).

106. A. Lifchez and A. Scommegna, Fertility and Sterility, 21, 426 (1970).

107. R. Schuhmann and H. D. Taubert, Acta Biol. Med. Germ., 24, 897 (1970).

108. V. Zbuzkova and F. A. Kincl, Steroids, 16, 447 (1970).

109. G. Benagiano and M. Ermini, Clin. Obstet. Gynec., 71, 51 (1969).

INFLUENCE OF PHYSICO-CHEMICAL PROPERTIES OF DRUG AND SYSTEM ON RELEASE OF DRUGS FROM INERT MATRICES

Gordon L. Flynn

University of Michigan

Ann Arbor, Michigan 48104

In designing chemical delivery systems or devices, one must optimize the rate of release of active ingredient so that the chemical agent is released in sufficient quantity to exert the desired biological effect while at the same time is released efficiently to assure protracted control with minimum biological or ecological side effects. There are many potential means of accomplishing these ends. The choice of the best system for a given use is highly dependent on the biological and chemical properties of the active compound and on its physico-chemical interactions in the system. I will attempt to thoroughly analyze one such system (the inert diffusional matrix) from these standpoints. Although the principles are general, my outlook is biased from my experiences with pharmaceutical systems.

I. GENERAL ANALYSIS OF MATRIX RELEASE

The term inert matrix needs definition. Inertness here implies a system insoluble in the in vivo setting; that is, a system which remains essentially intact throughout the period of drug release. This distinguishes it from active matrix systems which disintegrate or dissolve and, in the process, meter out active ingredient. Thus the inert matrix is a system in which drug release is totally dependent on passive diffusional processes. It should be pointed out that inertness also implies a high degree of biocompatibility.

The Type I Matrix

There are two distinct inert matrix systems which
have been characterized to a reasonably complete extent.
In one the matrix is formed by compressing a mixed granu-
lation of the active ingredient and an inert, relatively
impermeable solid diluent such as a wax or a deformable
plastic. Release from this system involves dissolution
of the drug directly into the external fluids bathing
the surface of the system. As the active ingredient is
eluted, external fluid is drawn into capillaries formed
in the matrix during the solution process. Release at
long time is by diffusion through these fluid-filled
spaces or capillaries to the outside of the matrix and
the bulk fluid. We can arbitrarily classify this as a
Type I device. The release mechanism for the Type I
device in terms of the total amount released in time, t,
is given[1] by Equation (1):

$$Q = \left[\frac{D\varepsilon}{\tau} (2W - C_s)C_s t \right]^{\frac{1}{2}} \tag{1}$$

where Q is the cumulative amount of substance released
per unit area of matrix surface, D is the effective diffusion coefficient of the drug in the solvent-filled
channels, ε is the porosity of the matrix, τ is the
tortuosity or degree of nonlinearity of the formed capillaries, W is the drug loading, C_s is the solubility
of the substance in the eluting solvent, and t is time.
By reason of its method of manufacture, which introduces
system limitations on factors such as size, shape, and
types of suitable materials, the Type I system is possibly of less importance than the Type II system to be
discussed. Therefore I will use the Type II matrix for
the prototype analysis.

The Type II-a Matrix

With regard to Type II matrices and drug delivery,
the release mechanism is diffusion of the active agent
through the matrix continuum rather than through formed
pores. Currently available examples of Type II systems
range from simple capped pieces of polymeric tubing
filled with active agent to molded polymeric devices
containing a significant volume fraction of suspended
drug. The drug release profile for such systems is
complex and is dependent on both drug-matrix and drug-
matrix-environment interactions.

Disregarding cylindrical geometrical considerations, the filled tube or "sausage" device becomes mechanistically a simple membrane transport situation. This system is schematically represented in Figure 1. When the core consists of excess suspended solid in a suitable fluid medium (possibly as a slurry or paste), release into a sink may be mathematically found by computing the total diffusional resistance from core to external media. [Note: A tube filled simply with solid drug is not considered, as the true area of drug-wall contact is uncertain and such devices thus behave erratically.] The total diffusional resistance is equal to the sum of the diffusional resistances encountered in the solvent diffusion layer in the core, in the membrane, and in the aqueous diffusion layer at the external surface.[2-4]

$$R_t = R_s + R_m + R_{aq} \tag{2}$$

Here R represents resistance and the subscripts t, s, m, and aq stand for total, solvent, membrane (or matrix), and aqueous, respectively. Since an individual diffusional resistance may be defined[3-4] by:

$$R_i = \frac{h_i}{D_i K} \tag{3}$$

where h_i is thickness, D_i is diffusivity in layer i of the laminate, and K is a partitioning term reflecting relative capacity for the diffusant, it follows that:

$$R_t = \frac{h_s}{D_s} + \frac{h_m}{D_m K_{m/s}} + \frac{h_{aq}}{D_{aq} K_{aq/s}} \tag{4}$$

where the partitioning terms are defined with respect to the initial phase encountered, the solvent (where $K_{s/s} = 1$). Under the conditions stated, diffusion into an infinite reservoir (sink) in the steady state is represented by flux expression:

$$\frac{dQ}{dt} = \frac{C_s}{R_t} \tag{5}$$

where the flux, dQ/dt, is equal to the driving force, C_s, which is the solubility in the "slurry" or internal solvent, divided by the total resistance. Therefore:

$$\frac{dQ}{dt} = \left[\frac{D_s D_m D_{aq} K_{m/s} K_{aq/s}}{h_s D_m D_{aq} K_{m/s} K_{aq/s} + h_m D_s D_{aq} K_{aq/s} + h_{aq} D_s D_m K_{m/s}} \right] C_s \tag{6}$$

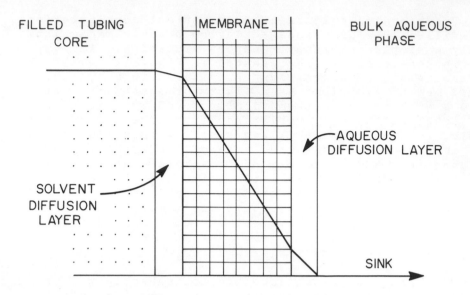

Figure 1.   Activity gradient through a filled tubing
            matrix system.

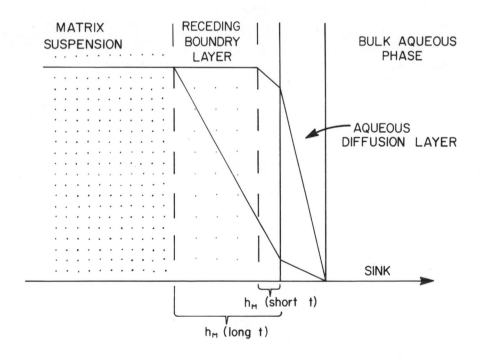

Figure 2.   Activity gradients at short and long times
            in a planar matrix release system.

Considering wall thicknesses of current devices and relative diffusivities between fluid and polymeric phases, one finds that usually $h_m D_s D_{aq} K_{aq/s} >> h_s D_m D_{aq} K_{m/s} K_{aq/s}$ + $h_{aq} D_s D_m K_{m/s}$ and the flux equation simplifies to:

$$\frac{dQ}{dt} = \left(\frac{D_m K_{m/s}}{h_m}\right) C_s \tag{7}$$

However, it is quite possible in view of the hydrophobic character of some of the drugs of interest that the value of K_{aq} can be sufficiently small or that K_m can be sufficiently large so that the aqueous boundary layers control the release. In this case the flux equation reduces to:

$$\frac{dQ}{dt} = \left(\frac{D_{aq} K_{aq/s}}{h_{aq}}\right) C_s = \left(\frac{D_{aq}}{h_{aq}}\right) C_{aq} \tag{8}$$

Note that the product of $K_{aq/s}$ and C_s yields the aqueous solubility of the diffusant, C_{aq}. It is unlikely unless a highly viscous solvent or an extremely poor solvent were employed in the core that the release would be controlled in the internal solvent diffusion layer.

The Type II-b Matrix

Equations for matrix release from systems where the drug is suspended in the continuum of the inert matrix were derived by T. Higuchi[5] and later generalized by Roseman and W. Higuchi[6]. Again, for simplicity of analysis, we will consider only the planar case depicted in Figure 2. Characteristic of these systems is a receding boundary of suspended drug as the drug is released from the system. Under the conditions that the total amount of drug in the matrix per unit volume, W, is much greater than the drug's matrix solubility, C_m; that a quasi-steady state exists; that the suspended particles are small relative to the distance of diffusion; and that the release is into a perfect sink; the following two equations collectively allow for characterization of release from this system:

$$h_m^2 + \frac{2 D_m h_{aq} h_m K}{D_{aq}} = \frac{2 D_m C_m}{W} t \tag{9}$$

and

$$Q = Wh_m \qquad (10)$$

For reasons which will become evident later, the matrix-water partition coefficient, K, in this case has been defined as the equilibrium concentration in the matrix over that in water rather than the reciprocal term found in the cited reference. The first equation, Equation (9), characterizes the thickness of the suspension depleted zone in the matrix with respect to time, and the second, Equation (10), defines the amount released as a function of this thickness. Two distinct dependencies are evident. When h_m is very small (initial conditions) or when K is very large, the term $2D_m h_{aq} h_m K/D_{aq} >> h_m^2$, and Equations (9) and (10) can be combined in this circumstance,

$$Q = \left(\frac{D_{aq} C_m}{K h_{aq}}\right) t \qquad (11)$$

Since $C_m/K = C_{aq}$, the aqueous solubility,

$$Q = \left(\frac{D_{aq}}{h_{aq}}\right) C_{aq} t \qquad (12)$$

Thus these equations state that initially, when h_m is very small, and for a prolonged period if K is large, release will be linear with time and controlled by the diffusion layer.

For a thick matrix h_m will eventually become sufficiently large so that $h_m^2 >> 2D_m h_{aq} h_m K/D_{aq}$. This condition defines a new release dependency, i.e.,

$$Q = (2WD_m C_m t)^{\frac{1}{2}} \qquad (13)$$

which is the familiar square root of time relationship of T. Higuchi.[5] In this case the controlling factor in release is diffusion across the matrix continuum's clear boundary layer with dissolution of the suspended drug particles at the receding boundary interface.

If one evaluates the flux, dQ/dt, from the Type II-b matrix as a function of time, a rather interesting profile, as shown in Figure 3, is obtained. Figure 3 indicates that there are two periods of relatively invariant

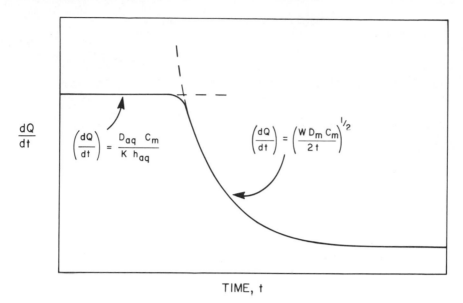

$$\frac{dQ}{dt}$$

$$\left(\frac{dQ}{dt}\right) = \frac{D_{aq}\ C_m}{K\ h_{aq}}$$

$$\left(\frac{dQ}{dt}\right) = \left(\frac{W\ D_m\ C_m}{2t}\right)^{1/2}$$

TIME, t

Figure 3.   Flux from a matrix as a function of time.

release rate, one at short t and one at long t.   In the
intervening period there is a mechanism change and a
dramatic drop in drug delivery rate.   Systems operating
essentially by diffusion layer control or systems which
rapidly become matrix controlled can be expected to meter
reasonably constant increments of drug to the release
site in a given period of time.

There are several additional variables which should
be introduced into the treatment of the Type II matrix
system.   In many if not most polymeric systems of interest, diffusionally impervious particles such as fillers
or polymeric crystallites are to be found in the matrix
continuum.   The preceding equations must then be adjusted
to account for: (1) the fractional cross-sectional area
occupied by these particles, and (2) the degree to which
distance along the flux vector is distorted and length-
ened by the presence of the particles.   Since the fractional cross-sectional area available for diffusion is
equivalent to the continuum volume fraction, V_1, the
continuum volume fraction is incorporated into the equation.   It should be recognized that $V_1 = (1 - V_2)$ where
V_2 is the filler volume fraction.   A tortuosity term, τ,
which is the ratio of the effective pathlength to the
shortest pathlength, accounts for the second effect and:

$$(\tau h_m)^2 + \frac{2D_m h_{aq}(\tau h_m)KV_1}{D_{aq}} = \frac{2D_m C_m}{W} t \qquad (14)$$

Adjustments to the filled tubing equations to account
for the same factors are obvious.

Examination of Equations (7), (8), and (14) reveals
that the Type II system variables, controllable and un-
controllable, are:

1. thickness of the unfilled zone in the
    matrix, h_m
2. matrix diffusivity, D_m (or membrane
    diffusivity)
3. aqueous diffusion layer thickness, h_{aq}
4. aqueous diffusivity, D_{aq}
5. the matrix/water partition coefficient, K
6. continuum solubility of the active ingre-
    dient, C_m
7. total amount of drug in the matrix per
    unit volume, W
8. the amount of filler which in turn deter-
    mines the values of V_1 and τ
9. although unexpressed, the overall
    geometrics of the system.

We can now analyze matrix release with respect to these
variables and, in particular, consider what might be
done to the permeant or system to alter the release
characteristics.

II. EFFECT OF SYSTEM VARIABLES ON MATRIX RELEASE

Diffusion Layer Variables

The properties of the boundary layer in the aqueous
phase post application of the matrix device are generally
not among the controllable variables of the system. With
the exception of geometrical considerations, such as cor-
rugating the matrix surface to increase the effective
thickness of the unstirred layer, diffusion layer thickness and diffusivity can be dismissed as manipulable
system variables.

Membrane Thickness, h_m

The thickness of the membrane, h_m, in the filled tubular system is an easily adjustable parameter and its manipulation provides virtually all the drug-delivery control one needs after a suitable membrane material and possibly supporting framework have been chosen for this system. In the matrix release system h_m is itself a variable and is sensitive to all other system parameters.

Matrix Diffusivity, D_m

One of the system parameters experiencing wide extremes of possible values is the membrane or matrix diffusion coefficient, D_m. At the outset one has a myriad of polymeric materials from which to choose for the matrix device. Diffusivities of drugs and drug-like substances in some of the materials that have been considered for drug-delivery systems vary a thousand-fold or more. Although highly practical considerations such as toxicity and biocompatibility reduce the number of materials to a small fraction of the total, there is still a broad range of polymeric materials to choose from and it is certain that new suitable materials are forthcoming.

It is perhaps more relevant and interesting to discuss means of manipulating diffusivity in a given polymer. In order to do this it is first necessary to consider what factors govern the diffusion of small molecules through a polymeric structure. This requires a little background in diffusion theory in liquids. In Figure 4 a two-dimensional diffusion field with a diffusing molecule identified as X is shown. Molecule X can change its equilibrium position in several ways. For instance X may obtain sufficient, timely kinetic energy to squeeze out of its solvent cage and move directly into a liquid void or "hole" large enough to accomodate it, as represented by the first mechanism in Figure 4, or it may revolve in concert with several other molecules, as depicted in the alternate mechanism in Figure 4, in each case to assume the same new equilibrium position. In either situation molecule X is said to have "jumped" to a new position and a "jump distance", δ, is assigned to the average such movement. Each of the mechanisms implicit in Figure 4 requires a considerable looseness of packing in the liquid state; otherwise the "jumps"

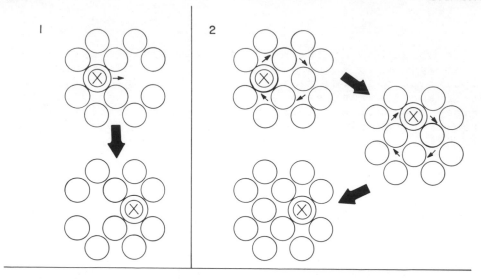

Figure 4.   Schematic representations of molecule X
            "jumping" into a new equilibrium position
            by void occupation (1) and by cooperative
            rotation (2).

would be highly restricted as in the solid state. The
"degree of looseness" is taken as the volume of the
liquid over and above that which the liquid would occupy
at the absolute zero of temperature and is called the
"free volume". From the dynamics of the liquid state
at the molecular level, it is obvious that X will change
its equilibrium position frequently. If it changes its
position ϕ times per second, where ϕ is the "jump
frequency"[7,8], then the diffusion coefficient can be defined by:

$$D = k\phi\delta^2 \tag{15}$$

where k is a constant (k = 1/6). It is thought unlikely
that the value of δ will vary much for X from liquid to
liquid and thus diffusivity differences between liquids
for X are largely attributed to the "jump frequency", ϕ.
The "jump frequency" it turns out is totally dependent
on the free volume or the looseness of the liquid structure. To be specific, the jump frequency is proportional
to the rate of hole formation of adequate size and proximity to X so that X can occupy it. It is assumed that
X will occupy all such holes as numerous molecular
oscillations of sufficient energy to propel X into a

hole occur during the lifetime of a hole. There are many
liquid properties responsive to the extent of free volume
in a liquid which can be used as a measure of the free
volume of a given system. One of these is viscosity and
a second is the temperature differential between the
experimental temperature and the liquid's glass-transition temperature. In the case of liquids the former is
most experimentally accessible and thus equations relating diffusivity to viscosity are widely used. The glassy
state of liquids is observed for few materials as most
liquids crystallize readily at temperatures considerably
above the glass-transition region.

The equation relating diffusivity to "jump distance"
and "frequency of jumps" is comparably pertinent to diffusion through a polymeric field.[7] In this case the
holes are formed by movements, singly and cooperatively,
of the basic polymeric units, which in many ways act as
small molecules. The probability of a polymeric unit or
segment assuming a new equilibrium position is therefore
also dependent on the "extent of looseness" or free volume
of the polymeric structure. The segmental "jump frequency" will also be influenced by other geometrical and
vibrational factors. However, as in the case of liquids,
these factors are not nearly so important as the free-
volume factor. In the case of polymers experimental
estimation of the molecular level viscosity is difficult
or impossible but glass-transition temperatures are
readily determined. So it is the differential between
experimental temperature and glass-transition temperature which provides the most practical assessment of the
molecular-level openness of the structure.

We can now consider what system-adjustable factors
affect diffusivity and by what mechanism. Some of these
factors are listed in Table I.

Table I. Factors which Influence Diffusivity
          in Polymers

Factor	Net influence on D_m
Increased polymer molecular weight	decrease
Increased degree of polymer crosslinking	decrease
Diluents and plasticizers	increase
Fillers	decrease
Increased crystallinity	decrease
Co-polymerization	either way

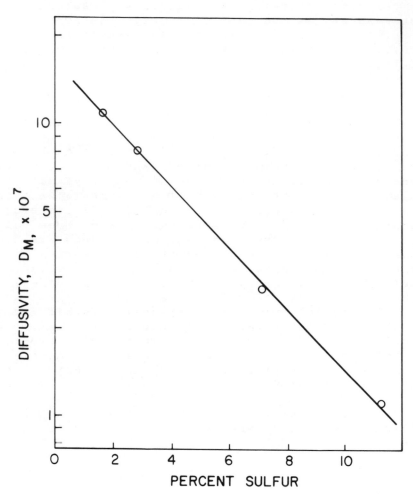

Figure 5.   Effect of crosslinking on diffusion of
            nitrogen through natural rubber at 25°C.

In the light of what was said about free volume and its relationship to glass-transition temperature, T_g, we can rationalize each of the tabulated effects with respect to its influence on T_g values. Not so incidentally, the glass-transition temperature is that temperature at which the molten polymer is transformed into a hard glass, in which, on the molecular level, the polymer has essentially lost its segmental mobility. This temperature is about 1/2 to 3/4 the value of the polymer's melting point, T_m, or point where polymeric crystallites are formed as temperature is lowered (on the absolute temperature scale). Just below the glass-transition temperature the free volume appears to be only 1/40 of the total volume for all glasses.

As average molecular weight of a polymer is increased, the glass-transition temperature is increased and thus diffusivity is decreased. This is because chain ends possess more free volume than segments pinned at both ends in the middle of the polymeric strand. The following relationship[7] has been shown to be applicable:

$$T_g = T_g^\infty - \frac{B}{M} \qquad (16)$$

where T_g^∞ is the glass-transition temperature at infinite chain length and B is a constant directly related to the number of chain ends per unit volume of polymer. The effect of reducing the average molecular weight, M, can be quite large. Polystyrene M = 3000 has a T_g of 45°C while polystyrene M = 300,000 has a value of 100°C. Considering that we might be more interested in increasing diffusivity than the reverse, then one should choose the lowest molecular-weight fraction of a polymer possible for a given purpose.

Adjusting the degree of crosslinking in a polymer represents another practical method of manipulating diffusivity. It has been found[8] as the degree of crosslinking increases, diffusion coefficients decrease. Barrer and Skirrow[9] have demonstrated this effect for the diffusion of nitrogen gas through natural rubber as a function of the degree of vulcanization. The diffusivities they obtained are plotted semilogarithmically against the percent of added crosslinking agent, in this case sulfur, in Figure 5. It is evident that diffusivity drops exponentially with crosslinking, at least for this system at 25°C. The effect of crosslinking has been shown to be more exaggerated for larger diffusing

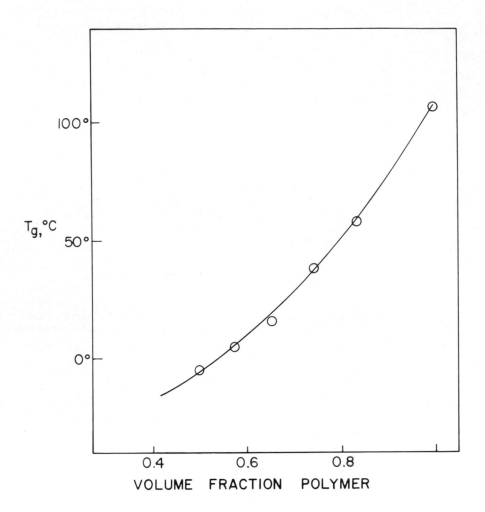

Figure 6. Effect of additive, diethyl phthalate, on
           glass transition of poly(methyl methacrylate).

species. Both the crosslinking effect itself and the
size dependency thereof are in accord with the hole
theory for diffusion. By pinning molecular segments together _via_ crosslinks, polymer flexibility is compromised
and hole formation rendered more difficult. It is
expected then that increased crosslinking will raise the
glass-transition temperature and this is indeed observed.
Therefore, if maximized diffusivity is desired, the
minimum extent of crosslinking of a polymer consistent
with the necessary mechanical properties to form a good
drug-delivery device should be sought. Moreover, one
might use the glass-transition point of a material as a
control check on the reproducibility of the crosslinking
process which will affect the ultimate performance of
the delivery system.

The role of polymeric plasticizers in "loosening up"
the polymeric matrix may in some instances provide a
means of adjusting diffusivity. Plasticizers and diluents
perform two functions which contribute to free volume.
At low concentrations the influence is primarily one of
reducing interchain interactions. In concentrations where
the additive can be considered a diluent, the free volume
of the diluent must be added to that of the polymer and a
net increase in free volume is experienced. As expected,
the glass-transition temperature is a highly sensitive index of this influence. This is illustrated in Figure 6
where the glass-transition temperature of poly(methyl
methacrylate) is shown as a function of the concentration
of plasticizer, diethyl phthalate.[10] Bueche[7] gives
expressions for quantitating this effect. It may be
concluded that plasticizers will accelerate the diffusive
process.

Fillers incorporated into a polymeric matrix decrease
diffusivity. The influence is largely due to the reduction of continuum volume fraction, V_1, and to tortuosity,
τ, as previously discussed. However, if the filler
particulates are sufficiently finely dispersed, they may
in effect become points of crosslinking _via_ physical
adsorption of polymeric strands, and this can potentially
have a profound effect on diffusivity as explained in
discussing chemical crosslinking. Generally fillers are
coarsely dispersed and the latter influence is not
particularly large. Other influences noted in membrane
transport experiments such as physical adsorption of diffusant[11-13] should not dramatically affect matrix release
profiles as the adsorption sites would be "saturated"
prior to administration of the device. In other words,
active fillers primarily influence the non-stationary

state. One must be careful however to consider this influence when determining diffusivities independently by
the membrane method; otherwise incorrect estimates of
matrix diffusivity, D_m, may be introduced into the matrix
release expression.

Like extremely finely dispersed filler particles,
crystallites act as physical crosslinks between chains
and, as such, reduce the net chain flexibility and corresponding diffusivity. Like fillers, they also act as
relatively impermeable physical obstacles in the path of
the diffusing species and require that one account for
continuum volume fraction, V_1, and tortuosity, τ, in the
matrix release equation. As one might expect, crosslinking is more important here than the latter mechanical
influences and those factors which suppress the crystal-
lization temperature, T_m, produce a comparable suppression of the glass-transition temperature, T_g. However,
it is possible to influence the nature of the crystallites formed and the degree of crystallite formation by
varying the polymeric processing method and such manipulation should markedly influence diffusivity in a
given system.

The random copolymer or sequentially altering copolymer also has promise with respect to diffusivity
adjustment. It is believed that the free volume of the
copolymer is a function of the individual free volumes
of the pure polymeric materials, which to a degree are
presumed additive. Bueche[7] has given this mathematical
expression. Wood[14] has experimentally demonstrated that,
at least qualitatively, this reasoning is sound. Thus
there is hope that experienced polymer chemists will be
able to tailor copolymers to the needs of the drug-
delivery system.

Absolute Matrix Solubility, C_m

One of the more important system variables in matrix
release is solubility of the active agent in the matrix
phase. This is a highly restricting parameter as it
should be remembered that in the matrix control situation
the release rate is proportional to the square root of
matrix solubility (Equation 13). There are two distinct
concerns regarding solubility: (1) what is the absolute
solubility of the drug of choice in the matrix of choice
and to what extent can this be manipulated; and (2) where
there are several compounds from which to choose, what

are the influences of chemical structural differences between analogs or homologs and how can these be used to
select the most appropriate compound with respect to drug
delivery?

The absolute solubility of a chemical in an amorphous
polymer is determined by the same factors which establish
solubility in liquids. This is a complex, thermodynami-
cally controlled equilibrium. Solute crystal energetics
are balanced against the free energy of mixing and other
enthalpic and entropic processes occurring in the solution process. Since most matrix materials suited to the
construction of delivery systems are relatively non-polar,
the solubility parameter concept of Hildebrand and Scott[15]
may be used to obtain a "ballpark" a priori estimation of
solubility. For example, in the case of alkyl-p-aminobenzoates, solubilities in liquid polydimethylsiloxane
were found to be similar to those in hexane and were
highly correlated with solubility parameter over a broad
range of chain length.[16] Of course actual solubility in
the matrix can be measured either kinetically[17] or by
equilibrium methods.[18]

There are a limited number of ways by which solubility
can actually be manipulated; all involve use of some high-
energy (meta-stable) crystal form. Thus polymorphs, high-
energy solvates and high-energy co-precipitates have real
promise in this regard. What is particularly attractive
is that the meta-stable highly soluble crystal forms may
be inhibited from reverting to the stable crystal form
when incorporated into the polymeric matrix. In other
words, the process of nucleation may be suppressed sufficiently so such forms can be utilized. Since other
matrix system parameters such as diffusivities and partition coefficients will not be influenced by the crystal
form employed, any real increase in solubility will be
experienced as a real increase in release rate, i.e., as
a direct ratio in diffusion layer control and as a square
root ratio in matrix control.

Compound selection may also involve matrix solubility
considerations. In general the compound with the best
combination of low melting point (low crystal energetics)
and greatest similarity in "polarity" to the matrix phase
will be the most soluble. Once one of the members of a
class of compounds has been characterized with respect to
solubility and its solubility parameter calculated by the
fitting technique illustrated by Yalkowsky and Flynn,[16]
relative solubilities of other similar compounds can be

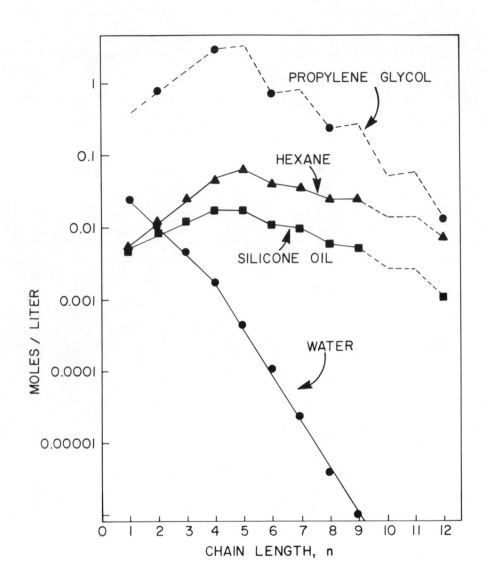

Figure 7.   Influence of alkyl chain length on solubility
            of p-aminobenzoates in some diverse solvents.

accurately estimated from solubility parameters obtained
by a functional group contribution approach.[16,19]   It
should be stressed that this applies to non-polar phases
only; solubility parameters are highly questionable where
hydrogen-bonding or, particularly, hydrophobic associa-
tions contribute to the free energy of solution.   To
illustrate these points consider the data in Figure 7
where the solubilities of the alkyl-p-aminobenzoates in
hexane, silicone oil, propylene glycol (even members
only) and water are plotted semilogarithmically against
chainlength, n.   When compared to melting points or heats
of fusion, it is found that the solubilities of these
homologs in the organic phases are highly responsive to
crystal energetics and thus it can be concluded that, in
these solvents, the crystal energetics play the dominant
role in determining the relative solid-solution equi-
libria insofar as chain length is concerned.   Note that
the solubilities in the organic solvents vary less than
fifty fold over the broad range of chain length exhibited
and that absolute solubility in a non-polar solvent such
as hexane is not necessarily increased as chain length is
extended (as some people generally assume).

     The aqueous solubility profile is remarkably dif-
ferent.   Odd-even alterations in solubility observed in
the organic solvents past C_4 chain length are masked
within the very large decreases in aqueous solubility
occurring as chain length is extended.   Aqueous solubilities from C_1 to C_9 chain length are spread over five
logarithmic orders.   The fact that there are two distinct slopes in the aqueous profile corresponding to
regions where the melting points are falling (up to C_4)
and then increasing indicates that crystal energetics
are still important.   However, it is also obvious that
there is another superimposed free energy factor of
greater significance determining the solubility trend.
This factor is unfavorable negative entropy resulting
from structuring of water at the low energy hydrocarbon
surface, so-called hydrophobic bonding or association.
The extent of hydrophobic association is proportional
to the molecule's hydrocarbon surface area.

                    Partition Coefficient, K

     Matrix/water partition coefficients among different
compounds for a given matrix release system exhibit the
widest extremes of values of any system parameter.   The
reasons for this should be apparent from the previous

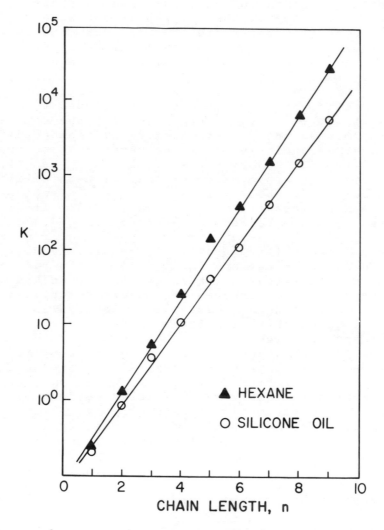

Figure 8.   Partitioning of alkyl p-aminobenzoates
            between oil and water.

discussion on absolute solubilities. By again considering the alkyl-p-aminobenzoates we can make some important
generalizations with respect to K and its influence on
the matrix release profile. In Figure 8 hexane/water and
silicone/water partition coefficients for this series are
displayed as a function of chain length. They increase
linearly on a semilogarithmic scale. Thus partitioning
follows the simple relationships:[4,20]

$$\log K_n = \log K_o + \pi n \qquad (17)$$

or

$$K_n = K_o 10^{\pi r} \qquad (18)$$

where K_n is the partition coefficient for the compound of
chain length, n, K_o is the Y intercept at zero chain
length and π is the slope for the semilogarithmic plot.
What is striking as we compare these data with the respective trends found for absolute solubilities is that
the partition coefficient function is not responding to
increasing "lipophilicity" of the compounds, but, obviously, to a dramatically increasing "hydrophobicity".
Free energy events in the aqueous phase are necessarily
dominant. Therefore it should not be so surprising that
π-values do not differ widely from one immiscible organic
phase to another.[21,22]

We can substitute the partitioning relationship
(Equation 18) into the matrix release equation to better
evaluate the partition coefficient influence. Combining
Equations (9) and (18) yields:

$$h_m^2 + \frac{2D_m h_{aq} h_m K_o 10^{\pi n}}{D_{aq}} = \frac{2D_m C_m}{W} t \qquad (19)$$

We will consider C_m, the matrix phase solubility, to be
relatively uninfluenced by increasing chain length. Examination of this equation and the exponentially growing
value of $10^{\pi n}$ and consideration of the circumstances
which lead to Equations (11) and (13) reveal that the
duration of the diffusion layer control period is extremely sensitive to alkyl chain length. All other
things being equal, release profiles in the form of the
log amount released at a given time, t_x, as a function of
chain length will appear as in Figure 9. As long as
$t_x \gg t_c$, where t_c is the critical time when the change
from diffusion layer control to matrix control occurs,

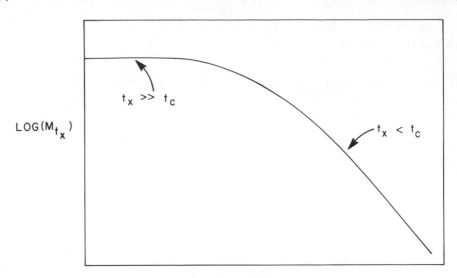

CHAIN LENGTH, n

Figure 9.   Influence of chain length on amount released
             at time t_x. Note that the point of mechanism
             change, t_c, is dependent on chain length.

the amount released at t_x will be invariant. However,
when $t_x < t_c$ the log (amount released) at t_x will drop
with a slope of $-\pi$. This will occur at long chain length
regardless of the choice of t_x. Another way this effect
can be seen graphically is to examine amount released
profiles as a function of time for different values of
n, as seen in Figure 10. Clearly, in the initial stages,
the matrix/water partition coefficient has a profound
effect on the drug delivery capabilities. Therefore,
if one can derivatize or by other means obtain compounds
with widely variant K without at the same time experiencing other counter productive changes (such as in C_m),
then one has a useful handle in designing an optimum
release profile.

The System Loading Factor, W

    One of the final variables to be considered is the
total amount of active ingredient incorporated in the
matrix per unit of matrix volume, W. This quantity and
the total volume of the device collectively yield the
device's total drug delivery capability. W also estab-
lishes the velocity of the receding boundary into the

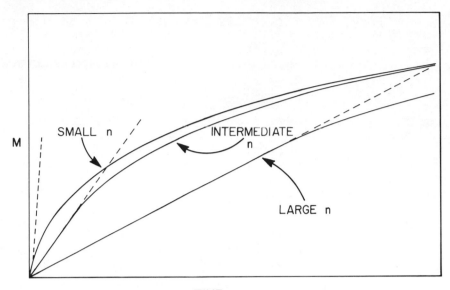

TIME, t

Figure 10.   Amount released, M, from matrix with time,
             as influenced by chain length, n.

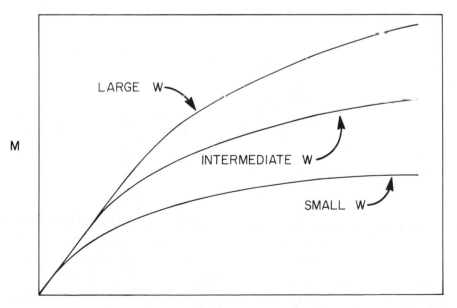

TIME, t

Figure 11.   Amount released, M, from matrix with time,
             as influenced by matrix loading, W.

matrix and thus, for a given system, it is a determinant
of both the duration of diffusion layer control and the
total amount released in time once matrix control is
operative. These effects are illustrated graphically in
Figure 11. It will be noted that the initial slopes -
that is, the initial flux from the matrix - is unaffected
by loading (the size of W). However, since at higher
loading the diffusion layer control period lasts longer
and the flux in matrix control is greater, the total
amount released eventually becomes quite sensitive to W.
Roseman and Higuchi[6] have neatly experimentally demonstrated this effect for medroxyprogesterone acetate released from a polydimethylsiloxane matrix.

                            Geometry

    There is one last system variable to mention in
passing, system geometry. The analysis here has dealt
only with release from a planar surface on a per-unit-
area basis. Obviously total release and the shape of
the release profile are also functions of size and shape
and other geometrics (like internal exposed surface) of
the matrix apparatus. Methods where the matrix surface
area is expanded or conserved, where device thickness is
increased or decreased, etc., need to be considered to
arrive at the optimum system for a given need.

    In conclusion, then, this analysis of the matrix re-
lease system indicates it has great system flexibility,
and manipulation of system performance parameters by
many practical, proven techniques is possible. There
are of course some inherent limitations to these systems
such as cost and the need for highly potent ingredients.
With these in mind, it should be possible to design and
construct useful and profitable delivery devices, devices
that comply with stringent a priori performance goals.

    One should not assume from the discussion of the dif-
ferential between glass transition and operating temperatures that glassy polymers are being considered. To the
contrary, amorphous polymers are best suited for most
drug-delivery purposes as they are pliable and diffusion
is relatively rapid through them. Increasing the rate
of release is more of a problem for these systems than
the reverse. What this differential does indicate,
albeit crudely, is the openness of the amorphous polymeric structure at ambient or physiological temperature.
Polymers tend to expand at comparable rates above their
glassy state.

It was pointed out in the conference that the glass-transition temperature is a second-order transition and as such cannot be precisely defined (it is sensitive to method and kinetics of measurement). However, it is important to note that a given method applied in a reproducible fashion will yield useful glass-transition values and differences will be real. So, the transition can be characterized in a practical way and serves as a useful index.

Lastly, data on diffusion of gases through polymers seem contradictory to the concepts presented. The concepts as presented of course do not apply to molecules sufficiently small to penetrate the polymer when its segments are static. Large molecules of interest, such as the steroids and pesticides, of course are too large to move with facility through a polymeric field unless the polymeric strands are capable of motions which can produce holes much greater in size than found in the "frozen" (glassy) state.

REFERENCES

1. T. Higuchi, J. Pharm. Sci., 52, 1145 (1963).

2. B. J. Zwolinski, H. Eyring, and C. E. Reese, J. Phys. Chem., 53, 1426 (1949).

3. R. J. Scheuplein, J. Theoret. Biol., 18, 72 (1968).

4. G. L. Flynn and S. H. Yalkowsky, J. Pharm. Sci., 61, 838 (1972).

5. T. Higuchi, J. Pharm. Sci., 50, 874 (1961).

6. T. J. Roseman and W. I. Higuchi, J. Pharm. Sci., 59, 353 (1970).

7. F. Bueche, "Physical Properties of Polymers," Interscience, N. Y., N. Y. (1962).

8. J. Crank and G. S. Park (Editors), "Diffusion in Polymers," Academic Press, N. Y., N. Y. (1969).

9. R. M. Barrer and G. Skirrow, J. Polymer Sci., 3, 549 (1948).

10. F. N. Kelley and F. Bueche, J. Polymer Sci., 50, 549 (1961).

11. W. I. Higuchi and T. Higuchi, J. Amer. Pharm. Sci., 49, 598 (1960).

12. C. F. Most, J. Appl. Poly. Sci., 14, 1019 (1970).

13. G. L. Flynn and T. J. Roseman, J. Pharm. Sci., 60, 1788 (1971).

14. L. A. Wood, J. Polymer Sci., 28, 319 (1958).

15. J. Hildebrand and R. L. Scott, "The Solubility of Nonelectrolytes," 3rd Ed., Rheinhold, N. Y., N. Y. (1950).

16. S. H. Yalkowsky, G. L. Flynn and T. G. Slunick, J. Pharm. Sci., 61, 852 (1972).

17. T. J. Roseman, J. Pharm. Sci., 61, 46 (1972).

18. R. J. Scheuplein, I. H. Blank, G. J. Brauner, and D. J. MacFarlane, J. Invest. Derm., 52, 63 (1969) and R. J. Scheuplein, J. Invest. Derm., 48, 334 (1965).

19. P. A. Small, J. Appl. Chem., 3, 71 (1953).

20. G. Saracco and E. S. Marchetti, Ann. Chem., 48 1357 (1958).

21. A. Leo, C. Hansch, and D. Elking, Chem. Rev., 71, 525 (1971).

22. S. H. Yalkowsky and G. L. Flynn, J. Pharm. Sci., 62, 210 (1973).

SILICONE RUBBER: A DRUG-DELIVERY SYSTEM FOR CONTRACEPTIVE STEROIDS

Theodore J. Roseman

The Upjohn Company

Kalamazoo, Michigan 49001

I. INTRODUCTION

Current methods for hormonal contraceptive therapy require that the drug be administered to the patient either orally or intramuscularly (as a suspension). Although efficacious, certain disadvantages exist with each route of administration. Oral administration necessitates the daily intake of a tablet and can result in undesirable side effects. Intramuscular administration of the steroid prevents conception for extended periods but is not immediately reversible. Newer methods of drug delivery are evolving which show promise in alleviating the undesirable aspects of the above modes of therapy.

In recent years much interest has been focused on the use of silicone rubber (polydimethylsiloxane) as a delivery system for contraceptive steroids. Hormonal-silicone devices have been tested, in animals and humans in the form of subcutaneous[1-5] or intrauterine[6-8] implants and vaginal rings.[9-10] The degree of success with each dosage form depends upon several factors such as the route of administration, the contraceptive agent employed, the design of the delivery system, and the desired duration of biological activity. Ideally, these systems deliver the drug either systemically or directly to the target organ in the minimal dose that is necessary to elicit the biological response. The dosage form, then, is considered to be programmed to release the drug at a reproducible and predetermined rate during the

course of treatment which can range from months to years.
The concept of sustained-release dosage forms is not new,
but as exemplified by the talks at this symposium, its
potential is virtually untapped.

In 1966, Dziuk and Cook[11] reported that several
steroids passed through the walls of silicone tubing.
In vitro as well as in vivo experiments demonstrated that
the steroids were released from the tubing for extended
time periods. Using progesterone as the test compound,
Kincl et al.[12] showed that its transport rate across a
silicone rubber membrane was orders of magnitude greater
than observed for other polymeric materials (Table I).
The high degree of tissue compatibility of silicone
rubber[13] combined with this excellent permeability
characteristic provides the basis for its use as a drug-
delivery system.

This paper is concerned with the use of silicone
rubber as matrix for the controlled release of contraceptive steroids. Special emphasis is given to the
mechanism of drug release and the factors which influence
the drug release process. In vitro and in vivo studies
using a vaginal device containing medroxyprogesterone
acetate provide the basis for the concepts which will be
developed throughout this paper. Physico-chemical principles are applied to provide quantitative mechanistic
interpretations of observed differences in release rates
of various steroids from the silicone matrix. Since
analogous concepts exist in membrane transport phenomena,
these are discussed in the appropriate sections.

Table I. Diffusion of ^{3}H Progesterone Through
Membranes of Various Polymers[12]

Polymer	Progesterone diffused, %
Polydimethylsiloxane (Silastic)	100
Acetylcellulose (Cellophane)	0.1
Fluoroethylene (Teflon)	0.1
Polyester (Mylar)	0.1
Polycarbonate (Lexan)	0.1
Polyethylene	0.1
Polyamide (Nylon)	1.0
Polystyrene copolymer (Cr39)	0.1

II. MECHANISM OF DRUG RELEASE

The mechanism of drug release from silicone polymers is based upon the diffusional process described by Fick's law.[14] From the physical model approach, mathematical equations are derived to describe the drug release process. These are dependent, however, upon the choice of the model system. Two types of silicone devices have been tested in biological systems and these are described below along with the appropriate relationships for the transport of drug across a silicone membrane.

Solid Suspension Model

Drug-silicone devices of the solid suspension type are prepared by encapsulating the drug in a polymeric environment.[15,16] The drug is incorporated into the monomers by levigation. The mix is catalyzed by the addition of catalyst and then placed into molds of the desired geometry. The device is removed from the mold after it is cured. In this model, the drug dissolves in the polymer and diffuses to the surface where it partitions into the aqueous environment. It then diffuses across an aqueous diffusion layer.

The following equations describe the release process for the general case where the transport of the drug is considered to occur across two planar regions, the matrix phase and the aqueous diffusion layer, which occur in series:[15]

$$Q = W\ell \qquad (1)$$

$$\ell^2 + \frac{2D_m h_a K \varepsilon \ell}{D_a \tau} = \frac{2D_m C_m \varepsilon t}{W\tau} \qquad (2)$$

where Q = amount released per unit area (mg/cm^2)
t = time (sec)
D_m = diffusion coefficient in the polymer (cm^2/sec)
D_a = aqueous diffusion coefficient (cm^2/sec)
C_m = solubility in the polymer phase (mg/cm^3)
K = partition coefficient (polymer/aqueous)
W = concentration of drug in the matrix (mg/cm^3)
τ = tortuosity
ε = volume fraction of the matrix
ℓ = diffusional distance (cm) in the polymer (zone of depletion)
h_a = diffusional distance (cm) in the boundary layer

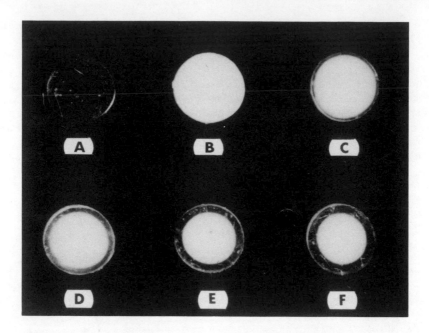

Figure 1.   Cross-sectional views of silicone (transparent)
            cylinders. Key: A = placebo; B = drug-filled
            initial; C = 1 week; D = 2 weeks; E = 3 weeks;
            F = 4 weeks.[15]

The mathematics for cylindrical geometry has also been
considered since devices in the form of cylinders and
rings have been used to a great extent. When the fraction of drug released is less than 50%, Equations (1)
and (2) can be used to approximate cylindrical geometry.[17]
As drug is released, a zone of depletion results (ℓ)
which increases with time as expected from Equation (2).
A photograph of these depletion zones is shown in Figure
1 for medroxyprogesterone acetate. Drug from the inner
core of the matrix travels across this zone, and the release rate decreases as a function of time in a predictable fashion.

     Consideration of the aqueous diffusion layer is an
extension of the Higuchi relationship[18] for the release
of drugs from matrix systems, as Equations (1) and (2)
reduce to the Higuchi equation

$$Q = \left(\frac{2WD_m C_m \varepsilon t}{\tau} \right)^{\frac{1}{2}} \qquad (3)$$

when $$\ell >> \frac{2D_m h_a K\epsilon}{D_a \tau}$$

When the above condition is not satisfied, matrix-diffu-
sion layer control (Equations 1 and 2) is operative and
Q versus $t^{\frac{1}{2}}$ is not linear at early times as predicted
by Equation (3). This is shown in Figures 2 and 3 where
the duration of the non-linear region is dependent upon
the progestational agent and its concentration respectively. The non-linear regions in Figure 2 are less
pronounced because of the expanded time axis. When
aqueous diffusion layer control is operative release
rates are less than expected from Equation (3) due to
the contribution of the second term in Equation (2).

Packed Tubing Model and Membrane Transport

Packed Tubing Model. A piece of silicone tubing of
the desired dimensions (wall thickness and length) is
packed with bulk drug crystals. The ends of the tubing
are sealed with a medical adhesive and the implant is
then sterilized. The drug in contact with the inside
wall of the tube dissolves in the polymer and diffuses
to the surface of the implant as described for the solid
suspension model. As drug is released, its reservoir
inside the tube is depleted. This results in settling
of packed drug and a concomitant reduction in drug contact with the interior walls of the tube. In this case,
the release of drug can be variable and unpredictably
low.[19-21] It has been suggested that uniform contact
can be achieved by suspending the drug within the capsule wall.[21] For this case, mathematical expressions
can be derived by analogy to the previous model.

Membrane Transport. Studies on the transport of
steroids, as well as other drug molecules, across silicone membranes have shown that permeability rates are
proportional to surface area and inversely proportional
to the thickness (x) of the membrane.[12,19,22-25] This
is illustrated by the following expression where diffusion through the membrane is rate controlling under
perfect sink conditions (concentration equals zero) on
the receptor side of the membrane.

$$\frac{dQ}{dt} = \frac{C_m D_m}{x} \qquad (4)$$

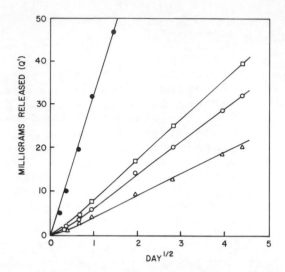

Figure 2.   Amount of steroid released from silicone
             cylinders as a function of the square root
             of time.   Key: ●, progesterone; □, medroxy-
             progesterone acetate; ○, 6α-methyl-11β-
             hydroxyprogesterone; and △, 17α-hydroxy-
             progesterone.[17] (Note that Q' is the amount
             released per cylinder).

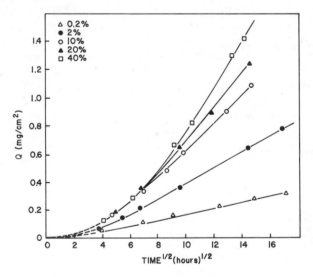

Figure 3.   Release of chlormadinone acetate (micronized)
             from silicone matrices as a function of the
             square root of time for several matrix con-
             centrations.[16]

Table II.   Average Diffusion Rate of Various
            Steroids Across Polydimethyl-
            siloxane Membrane[12]

Steroid	Diffusion rate μg[a]
19-Norprogesterone	1353
Progesterone	469
Testosterone	317
Megestrol acetate	236
Norethindrone	73
Estradiol	61
Mestranol	43
Corticosterone	21
Cortisol	6

a.   Diffusion rate: 100 mm^2/0.1 mm/24 hr.

It is also assumed that the solute is maintained at its
equilibrium solubility value on the donor side of the
membrane. The steady-state rate is achieved after a
finite time (lag time) which is equal[26] to $x^2/6D_m$. The
influence of the diffusion layer on the overall transport process is discussed below.

III.   FACTORS INFLUENCING RELEASE RATES

The rate of diffusion of steroids from silicone rubber matrices or across silicone rubber membranes is influenced by the structure of the steroid[11,17,19,27,28]
as shown in Table II. Transport rates are dependent
upon the degree of lipophilicity of the steroid. Those
with higher silicone solubilities generally exhibit
faster release rates,[27] as suggested by the equations.
For steroids which exhibit high membrane permeability
constants (product of KD_m), transport rates usually are
under diffusion layer control.[29] The degree to which
the diffusion layer influences the release process depends upon the thickness of the membrane and the stirring
conditions. This is illustrated by the following steady-
state expression derived for perfect sink conditions:

$$\frac{dQ}{dt} = \frac{C_m D_m D_a}{KD_m(h_1 + h_2) + D_a x} \qquad (5)$$

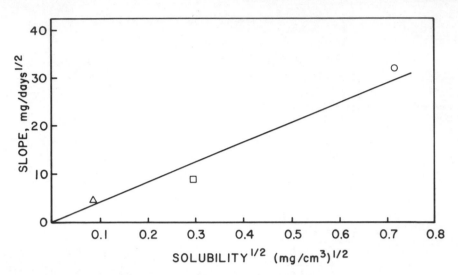

Figure 4.   Slope of Q' versus $t^{\frac{1}{2}}$ plots versus the square
             root of the solubility of the steroid in the
             silicone polymer.[17]   Key: ◯, progesterone;
             ▢, medroxyprogesterone acetate; and △,
             17α-hydroxyprogesterone.

where h_1 and h_2 are the diffusion layer thicknesses on
the donor and receptor side of the membrane respectively.
Smaller h values are experienced at faster stirring
speeds and Equation (5) reduces to Equation (4) when
$D_ax >> KD_m$ $(h_1 + h_2)$.

     In the case of the solid suspension model, the effect
of the diffusion layer on Q versus $t^{\frac{1}{2}}$ plots has already
been presented. For this model, slopes of Q versus $t^{\frac{1}{2}}$
plots are linearly dependent upon $(C_m)^{\frac{1}{2}}$ when matrix control is operative (Figure 4). The release profiles also
depend upon the concentration of drug within the matrix
as shown in Figures 5 and 6 for chlormadinone acetate and
medroxyprogesterone acetate respectively. The initial
release rates decrease as a function of time due to an
increased diffusional path within the matrix. At high
loading doses, this decrease is minimized.

     The effect of diffusion coefficients on the release
rate is evident from the equations. Diffusion coefficients for progestin-type steroids in polydimethylsiloxane
are approximately 5×10^{-7} cm^2/sec.[17] This value can be
orders of magnitude greater than diffusion coefficients

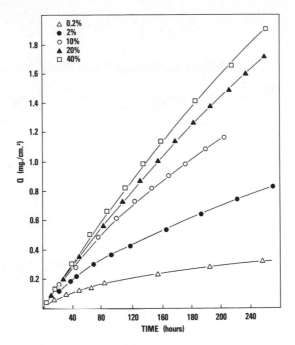

Figure 5.   Release of chlormadinone acetate (micronized)
            from silicone matrices as a function of time
            for several matrix concentrations.[16]

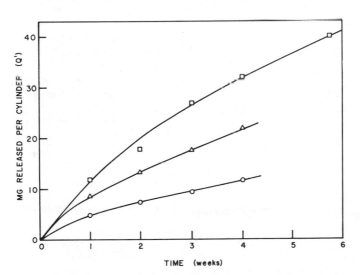

Figure 6.   Total amount of medroxyprogesterone acetate
            released from silicone cylinders as a function
            of time for three concentrations.[15]   Key:
            O = 3.0%; △ = 12.0%; □ = 24.0%.

Table III.   Permeability Constants of Three Steroids[33]
              Through Polysiloxane Membranes

Polysiloxane membrane	Permeability constant $\mu g/cm^2/hr$ $(x\ 10^{-4})$		
	Norprogesterone	Dehydro-cortisol	Cortisol
Dimethyl	659±28.1	0.4±0.01	0.2±0.02
Methylphenyl	580±33.3	1.1±0.04	0.6±0.05
Trifluoro-propylmethyl	76.7± 5.1	*	0.06±0.002

*Not determined.

reported for smaller molecules in polyethylene.[30]   These
relatively high diffusion coefficients may be attributed
to the ease of hole formation for the diffusing species
resulting from the high segmental chain mobility within
the polymer.[31]

    Silicone rubber generally contains reinforcing silica
to give mechanical strength to the polymer. These filler
particles can decrease transport rates by providing a
more tortuous diffusional path for the drug molecule and
by decreasing the volume fraction of the matrix as illus-
strated by Equations (1) and (2). Just as important, adsorption of drug onto the filler will increase the time
to reach the steady state transport rate.[25,32]   The
presence of filler particles will also cause determined
partition coefficients to be overestimated and diffusion
coefficients to be underestimated.[17,32]

    The structure of the silicone rubber also alters
transport rates[33] as indicated in Table III.   The factors
responsible for these results were not elucidated but,
based upon the preceding discussion, changes in the diffusivity and/or solubility of the steroid in the membrane
phase could account for these findings.

IV.   IN VITRO - IN VIVO CORRELATIONS

    In vitro - in vivo correlations have been hampered by
the lack of a uniform in vitro dissolution apparatus and
variations in the steroid-silicone delivery system which
have been utilized, i.e., subcutaneous implants, intrauterine capsules and vaginal rings. In the packed tubing

model, severe constraints are placed on such correlations because the true area of contact of drug within the interior of the capsule wall can change as a function of time. Another complicating factor is that some in vitro release rate studies have been performed in closed systems thereby allowing the concentration of the steroid to approach its equilibrium solubility value. This restricts dissolution rates, as the driving force (concentration difference) for dissolution is diminished. In vitro permeability rates have been shown to follow Fick's law under non-perfect sink conditions,[19] but the relationship of these experiments to the in vivo situation is not clear. In fact, Schuhmann and Taubert[28] found higher in vivo release rates, presumably because in vitro studies were not performed under ideal sink conditions.

In vitro - in vivo correlations are needed to assist in the design of programmed drug-delivery systems and to provide information on the bioavailability of the drug molecule. Therefore, reasons for decreased in vivo release rates have been sought with the following being proposed:[20,21]

(a) walling off of the implant due to encapsulation by fibrous connective tissue
(b) effect of the site of implantation
(c) absorption of lipid components from the tissue into the device.

In addition, transport away from the surface of the implant across an aqueous diffusion layer could restrict the release process. The importance of the aqueous diffusion layer in controlling absorption has been demonstrated in certain biological systems,[34,35] and it has been suggested that it can influence the observed in vivo release pattern of medroxyprogesterone acetate (MPA) from vaginal rings.[15] If it is assumed that drug is removed from the absorption site as it is released from the device (the body acting as a perfect sink), then the Equations (1) and (2) can be utilized to describe the in vivo release pattern. Since the location of the vaginal ring is reproducible and its short residence time should result in no walling off, it provides an excellent model to test the diffusion layer concept.* It was previously

---

*There are no data to suggest that the absorption of lipids into the ring alters release rates.

Table IV.   Average Amount (Mg) of Medroxyprogesterone
            Acetate Released from 65 mm Vaginal Devices
            Per Cycle[10]

Cycle	16 Day	21 Day
1	23.2±2.2	29.0±3.6
2	22.8±3.4	27.8±3.7
3	19.7±5.0	27.5±2.6
4	21.5±3.3	25.9±2.8
5	19.5±4.1	27.5±3.5
6	20.2±3.5	26.1±1.7
Mean	21.2 mg	27.3 mg

demonstrated that these devices effectively inhibit ovu-
lation in humans at dose levels of less than one mg per
day;[10] and hence, this delivery system offers potential
as a method of contraceptive therapy.

Figure 7 shows the influence of the diffusion layer
thickness on the release profile of medroxyprogesterone
acetate from a silicone vaginal ring. At a value of
approximately 500 μ, the amount released is in reasonable
agreement with the in vivo loss of drug from the devices
(Table IV). Although other parameters* in Equation (2)
may be altered in the in vivo situation, analysis using
the aqueous diffusion layer provides a reasonable self-
consistent physico-chemical explanation for the approximate two-fold decrease in the amount released after 21
days in vivo. It is worth noting that stagnant layer
thicknesses of 250-500 μ were also estimated in in situ
intestinal absorption studies.[36] The fact[5] that doubling
the wall thickness of silicone capsules which contained
progestins decreased diffusion rates by only 10-30% is
consistent with the above concepts. For at large h_a
values, the contribution of the wall thickness becomes
less significant for those steroids which have high
permeability constants.

In order to further test the above diffusional concepts which were used to describe the drug release pro-

*Note that the value of D_a in Equation (2) is the expected
value in a dilute aqueous solution. The true D_a value in
the vaginal secretions may be lower due to a viscosity
increase. This would have the same effect as increasing
h_a, since D_a is in the denominator in Equation (2).

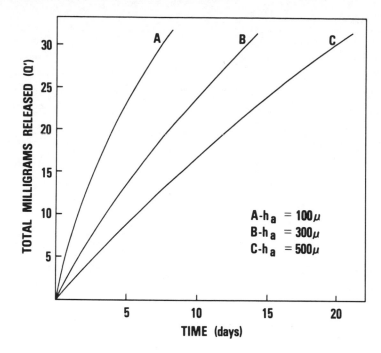

Figure 7. Theoretical profiles of the cumulative amount
of medroxyprogesterone acetate released from
vaginal devices as a function of time for
different diffusion layer thicknesses.

file, progesterone vaginal devices were evaluated in the
rhesus monkey. Figure 8 shows that peripheral plasma
levels after vaginal insertion of a 10 and 30% progesterone ring. Drug from the 2% ring was depleted as indicated
by low progesterone levels at 15-18 days post insertion.
In this study, progesterone was also released at a slower
in vivo rate as suggested by estimates of release rates
from the model.[37] In contrast, Sawardeker et al.,[38]
found that in vitro release rates of a non-steroidal drug
(2-methyl-3-ethyl-4-phenyl-4-cyclohexene carboxylic acid)
were in good agreement with in vivo availability in the
rhesus monkey. In this case, diffusion through the silicone tubing may have been the rate controlling step in
the absorption process.

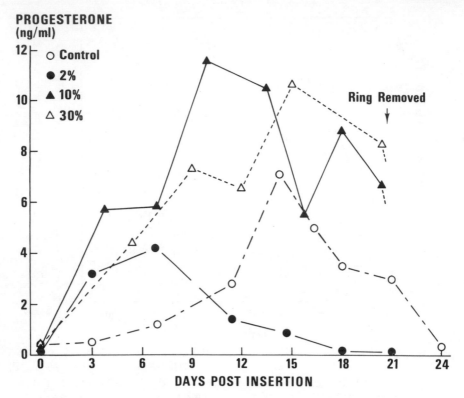

Figure 8.   Peripheral plasma progesterone concentrations
            in Rhesus monkeys with placebo or progesterone
            silicone vaginal devices.[37]

V.   SUMMARY

Silicone rubber (polydimethylsiloxane) was utilized
as a matrix for the controlled release of contraceptive
steroids. Hormonal devices can be prepared by either
suspending drug in the matrix phase or by packing the
steroid in tubing. A description of these two methods
of drug-delivery is presented.

The mechanism of drug release from such devices is
based upon Fick's law of diffusion. Depending upon the
choice of the model system, different mathematical relationships were presented to describe the drug release
process. Differences in _in vitro_ and _in vivo_ release
data can be related to changes in diffusion layer thickness. The influence of other physico-chemical parameters
on the drug transport process is also discussed.

ACKNOWLEDGMENT

Thanks are given to Dr. S. H. Yalkowsky for his helpful comments on the manuscript.

REFERENCES

1. H. Croxatto, S. Diaz, R. Vera, M. Etchart, and P. Atria, Amer. J. Obstet. Gynecol., 105, 1135 (1969) and Contraception, 4, 155 (1971).

2. H. J. Tatum, E. M. Coutinho, J. A. Filho, A. R. S. Sant'Anna, Amer. J. Obstet. Gynecol., 105, 1139 (1969).

3. E. M. Coutinho, C. E. R. Mattos, A. R. S. Sant'Anna, J. A. Filho, M. C. Silva, and H. J. Tatum, Contraception, 2, 313 (1970).

4. C. C. Chang and F. A. Kincl, Fertil. Steril., 21, 134 (1970).

5. A. S. Lifchez and A. Scommegna, ibid., 21, 426 (1970).

6. A. Scommegna, G. N. Pandya, M. Christ, A. W. Lee, and M. R. Cohen, ibid., 21, 201 (1970).

7. B. H. Vickery, G. I. Erickson, J. P. Bennett, N. S. Mueller, and J. K. Haleblian, Bio. Reprod., 3 154 (1970).

8. Y. Gibor, B. Seshadri, and A. Scommegna, Fertil. Steril., 22, 671 (1971).

9. D. R. Mishell, Jr., and M. E. Lumkin, ibid., 21, 99 (1970).

10. D. R. Mishell, Jr., M. E. Lumkin, and S. Stone, Amer. J. Obstet. Gynecol., 113, 927 (1972).

11. P. J. Dziuk and B. Cook, Endocrinology, 78, 208 (1966).

12. F. A. Kincl, G. Benagiano, and I. Angee, Steroids, 11, 673 (1968).

13. S. Braley, Ann. N. Y. Acad. Sci., 146, 148 (1968).

14. M. H. Jacobs, "Diffusion Processes," Springer-Verlag, New York, Inc. (1967).

15. T. J. Roseman and W. I. Higuchi, J. Pharm. Sci., 59, 353 (1970).

16. J. Haleblian, R. Runkel, N. Mueller, J. Christopherson, and K. Ng, ibid., 60, 541 (1971).

17. T. J. Roseman, ibid., 61, 46 (1972).

18. T. Higuchi, ibid., 52, 1145 (1963).

19. P. Kratochvil, G. Benagiano, and F. A. Kincl, Steroids, 15, 505 (1970).

20. E. Diczfalusy and U. Borell, eds., Nobel Symposium 15 "Control of Human Fertility," Wiley Interscience Division, New York, 1971, p. 46.

21. F. A. Kincl and H. W. Rudel, Acta. Endocrinologica - Suppl. 151, p. 5 (1971).

22. E. R. Garrett and P. B. Chemburkar, J. Pharm. Sci., 57, 944 (1968).

23. E. R. Garrett and P. B. Chemburkar, ibid., 57, 949 (1968).

24. E. R. Garrett and P. B. Chemburkar, ibid., 57, 1401 (1968).

25. G. L. Flynn and T. J. Roseman, ibid., 60, 1788 (1971).

26. R. M. Barrer, Trans. Faraday Soc., 35, 628 (1939).

27. K. Sundaram and F. A. Kincl, Steroids, 12, 517 (1968).

28. R. Schuhmann and H. D. Taubert, Acta. Biologica et Medica Germanica, 24, 897 (1970).

29. G. L. Flynn, O. S. Carpenter, and S. H. Yalkowsky, J. Pharm. Sci., 61, 312 (1972).

30. M. A. Gonzales, J. Nematollahi, W. L. Guess, and J. Autian, ibid., 56, 1288 (1967).

31. J. Crank and G. S. Park, "Diffusion in Polymers," Academic Press, New York, N. Y., 1968, pp. 54-58.

32. C. F. Most, J. Appl. Polym. Sci., 14, 1019 (1970).

33. S. Friedman, S. S. Koide, and F. A. Kincl, Steroids, 15, 679 (1970).

34. F. A. Wilson, V. L. Sallee, and J. M. Dietschy, Science, 174, 1031 (1971).

35. N. F. Ho and W. I. Higuchi, J. Pharm. Sci., 60, 537 (1971).

36. N. F. Ho, APhA Acad. of Pharm. Sci., Abstract Book 2, No. 2, 112 (1972).

37. K. T. Kirton, T. J. Roseman, and A. D. Forbes, Contraception, 8, 561 (1973).

38. J. S. Sawardeker, R. Gural, and J. McShefferty, APhA Acad. Pharm. Sci., Abstract Book 1, No. 1, 89 (1971).

FACTORS AFFECTING THE RELEASE OF STEROIDS FROM SILICONES

R. E. Lacey and D. R. Cowsar

Southern Research Institute

Birmingham, Alabama   35205

I.   INTRODUCTION

This paper describes research on factors that affect diffusion of steroids through siloxane polymers.
The research was undertaken to provide data needed for
the systematic development of improved contraceptive systems consisting of combinations of contraceptive steroids
and polymers to control the delivery of a steroid to a
target organ. Prior work on such controlled-delivery
systems has shown that long-term fertility control can
be achieved either by subcutaneous implants or by intravaginal or intrauterine devices. The prior research
also indicated fewer undesirable side reactions occur
with such systems than with oral administration of the
steroid. In the controlled-delivery systems studied
previously, dosage rates were maintained at a desired
level by controlling the rate of diffusion of steroids
from the steroid-polymer systems.

It has been demonstrated that the diffusion rates
from controlled-delivery systems follow Fick's second
law of diffusion, which states that the rate of diffusion
depends on five factors. Two of the factors involve the
dimensions of a device and three involve drug-polymer
interactions. The dimensional factors are the surface
area and the thickness through which diffusion occurs.
The three factors that are characteristic of each particular drug-polymer system are: the equilibrium solubility
of a drug in a polymer, C_m; the diffusivity of a drug in
a polymer, D; and the partition coefficient, K, of a drug

between the polymer and an external phase. With only a
few exceptions basic data have not been determined for
these last three factors, C_m, D, and K, that are needed
for the design of controlled-release devices. The research reported here is aimed toward obtaining the
needed data.

II. PERTINENT PRIOR RESEARCH

In 1966 Dziuk and Cook[1] showed that implants of contraceptive steroids (estradiol, progesterone, and others)
in capsules made of polydimethylsiloxane (PDMS) were effective in synchronizing estrous cycles in sheep. Their
use of PDMS with steroids stemmed from the earlier research of Folkman and Long[2,3] with anesthetic gases and
other agents, which permeated PDMS in biologically effective amounts; of Bass, Purdon, and Wiley[4] with
atropine and histamine, which were delivered at controlled rates from PDMS implants; and of Powers[5] with
antimalarial agents and antischistosomal drugs.

Segal[6] was the first to suggest the use of PDMS for
a long-lasting implant to control fertility in humans.

Following his suggestion, many studies were made
both in vitro and in vivo to explore the possibility of
a long-lasting contraceptive device. Garrett and
Chemburkar[7,8] studied the diffusion of a number of drugs
including progesterone through different polymeric membranes in vitro. They found membranes made of nylon and
cellulose esters to be almost impermeable but PDMS to be
permeable to progesterone. Kincl, Benagiano, and Angee[9]
found that the permeation rate of progesterone through
PDMS was 100 to 1000 times faster than the rates through
seven other polymers they studied. These workers also
found that the diffusion rates of various steroids
through PDMS differed markedly.

Sundaram and Kincl[10] showed that the rate of diffusion of a steroid through PDMS was directly proportional
to the area and inversely proportional to the thickness
of the membrane through which diffusion occurred, and
that the solubility of steroids in PDMS influenced diffusion rates. Kratochvil, Benagiano, and Kincl,[11] and
Friedman, Koide, and Kincl[12] showed that the transfer of
steroids through PDMS could be described by Fick's law
of diffusion.

If a drug is suspended in a fluid in contact with one side of a diffusion-controlling membrane and allowed to diffuse through the membrane into a different fluid, as occurs in one type of controlled-release contraceptive system, Fick's law is usually expressed in terms of the diffusion coefficient of the drug in the membrane, the appropriate partition coefficients, the concentrations of drug dissolved in the two fluids, the area of the membrane, and the thickness of the membrane.

$$\frac{dM}{dt} = \frac{DA(K_1 C_1 - K_2 C_2)}{h} \qquad (1)$$

where: $\frac{dM}{dt}$ = rate of diffusion of the drug through the membrane, $g\ sec^{-1}$

D = diffusion coefficient of the drug in the membrane, $cm^2\ sec^{-1}$

K_1 = partition coefficient of the drug between the suspending fluid and the membrane

C_1 - concentration of the drug dissolved in the suspending fluid, $g\ cm^{-3}$

K_2 - partition coefficient of the drug between the receptor fluid and the membrane

C_2 - concentration of the drug in the receptor fluid, $g\ cm^{-3}$

A = area of membrane, cm^2

h = thickness of membrane, cm

In controlled-release devices employing a suspending fluid the presence of undissolved drug in the donor fluid maintains the concentration of dissolved drug at the saturation level. The partition coefficient, K, is defined to be the ratio of the concentration of drug in the membrane to the concentration in the suspending fluid.

$$K = \frac{conc.\ of\ drug\ in\ membrane,\ g\ cm^{-3}}{conc.\ of\ drug\ in\ fluid,\ g\ cm^{-3}} \qquad (2)$$

The product, KC, is the concentration of drug in the membrane at the interface between membrane and suspending fluid. Since the concentration of drug in the suspending fluid is the saturation value, the interfacial concentration in the membrane, KC is also constant.

The drug diffusing through the membrane encounters resistance to transfer. The diffusion coefficient, which is a conductance term, is an inverse measure of the resistance the membrane offers to transfer of the drug. Polymers with high interchain attractions, high crosslinking densities, or strong interactions between moieties of the polymer chains and moieties on the transferring species offer high resistances to movement of drug molecules. Thus, the diffusion coefficient is low for such polymers.

When drug molecules have diffused to the side of the membrane opposite the suspending fluid, the molecules partition between the membrane and fluid in contact with that side. If the concentration of drug in this receptor fluid is C_2 at the membrane interface, the concentration within the membrane is K_2C_2 at that interface. A linear concentration gradient is formed within a homogenous membrane equal to

$$\frac{K_1C_1 - K_2C_2}{h}$$

In other types of controlled-release devices, powders of solid steroid are in contact with one side of a controlling membrane. Drug dissolves directly from the solid into the membrane, diffuses through the membrane, and is partitioned between the membrane and the receptor fluid.

For devices of this type the appropriate expression of Fick's law is

$$\frac{dM}{dt} = \frac{DA(C_m - K_2C_2)}{h} \tag{3}$$

where: C_m = equilibrium solubility of drug in membrane, $g\ cm^{-3}$

and the other terms have been defined previously.

It can be shown that for the first type of controlled-release device the concentration of drug within the membrane at the donor interface will be the equilibrium solubility, C_m, as long as solid steroid is present in the suspending fluids.

In controlled-release systems that use suspending fluids there will be an equilibrium between the solid drug and drug in solution, so the activity of the solid drug equals the activity of the drug in solution.

$$\frac{\text{activity of}}{\text{solid drug}} = \frac{\text{activity of drug}}{\text{in solution}} \qquad (4)$$

There will also be an equilibrium between drug dissolved in the fluid and drug dissolved in the membrane, so these two activities are equal.

$$\frac{\text{activity of drug}}{\text{in solution}} = \frac{\text{activity of drug}}{\text{in membrane}} \qquad (5)$$

Thus, at equilibrium, the activity of solid drug is equal to the activity of drug in solution, which in turn is equal to the activity of drug in the membrane.

Diffusion coefficients can also be calculated by the so-called time-lag equation, derived by Daynes[13] and generalized by Barrer.[14]

$$D = \frac{h^2}{6t_\ell} \qquad (6)$$

where: D = diffusion coefficient, cm^2 sec^{-1}

h = membrane thickness, cm

t_ℓ = the lag time, sec

From the data obtained in a typical diffusion experiment a graph of amount of steroid diffused versus time is prepared. A typical diffusion curve, as shown in Figure 1, is characterized by a portion in which only small amounts of steroid are diffused followed by a portion of the curve in which the rate of diffusion increases until a steady rate is reached (the straight-line portion to the right in Figure 1). This general shape of curve is predicted by the mathematical expressions derived by Daynes and Barrer. Extrapolation of the straight-line portion to the X-axis gives a value of the time lag (where the amount diffused equals zero).

The time lag can be interpreted as the time needed for the first diffusing molecules to be transported across the thickness of the diffusion barrier (i.e. membrane in these cases). Thus, the time-lag value of D calculated by the equation given should not be influenced by the resistance of diffusive boundary layers.

In addition to the above-cited work that bears directly on diffusion-control of drug delivery, there

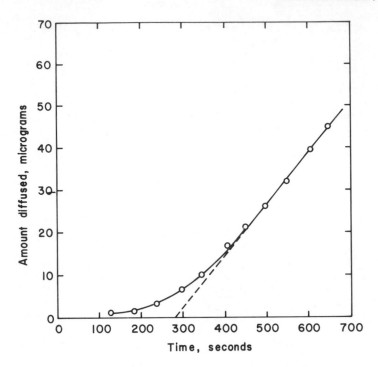

Figure 1.   Typical diffusion curve.

are a number of studies that show the efficacy of fertility control by the use of controlled-delivery systems.

Lifchez and Scommegna[15] showed that fertility could
be controlled in human volunteers with intrauterine devices in which contraceptive steroids were contained in
hollow cylinders made of PDMS. They also measured the
release rates of steroids in vivo from hollow-cylinder
devices implanted subcutaneously in rats. They found
the release rates in vivo (31.58 µg/day per mm of length)
were about three times the rates predicted from data
obtained by Kincl, Benagiano, and Angee[9] in vitro with
water as the receiving fluid, but corresponded well with
data obtained by Sundaram and Kincl[10] in vitro with re-
constituted human plasma as the receiving fluid (26.35
µg/day per mm of length). The difference between the
rates given by the two groups of workers was undoubtedly
due to a difference in partitioning between the membrane-
water and the membrane-plasma systems.

Mishell and his co-workers[16,17] studied the use of
intravaginal devices for administration of contraceptive
drugs. The devices were shaped like the outer ring of a

conventional contraceptive diaphragm (a toroid), and were
made of PDMS filled with crystals of a steroid. Mishell
found them to be both effective and convenient to use.
Roseman and Higuchi[18] developed mathematical expressions
to describe delivery rates from PDMS in which solid
steroid particles are uniformly dispersed, and verified
their expressions with experiments performed in vitro.
Their expressions included the effect of diffusional
boundary layers at the outside surfaces of the devices.
They showed that if a boundary-layer thickness of 580
microns were assumed as a "fitting-factor", the release
rates predicted by their mathematical expressions agreed
well with the release rates found by Mishell in his in
vivo experiments.

Clinical studies with human volunteers have been
made with subcutaneously implanted PDMS hollow-cylinder
devices containing megestrol acetate.[19,20] These
studies, which cover more than 800 woman-months, showed
about 75 to 110 µg/day of megestrol acetate delivered
from the implants to be effective for control of fertility.

Administration of contraceptive steroids from controlled-delivery devices thus promises to be an efficacious and convenient method of controlling fertility.
The delivery rates from the devices are controlled to
desired dosage rates by controlling the rate of diffusion
through the polymeric portions of the devices. In previous studies much attention has been given to the overall
diffusion rates (dM/dt), but data are needed on equilibrium solubilities, diffusion coefficients, and partition
coefficients for various steroids and different polymers,
so that design of the devices can proceed systematically.

III. EFFECTS OF STRUCTURES OF DRUGS AND MORPHOLOGY
      OF POLYMERS ON SOLUBILITY AND DIFFUSIVITY

In Section II the diffusion of steroids through
PDMS was shown to follow Fick's law. In Table I, the
data obtained by Kincl, Benagiano, and Angee[9] reveal
large differences in diffusion rates of different
steroids through PDMS. Since the data in Table I were
normalized for membrane area and thickness, the differences in rates must be related to differences in
solubilities, diffusion coefficients, or partition
coefficients, or all three.

Table I.   Diffusion Rates of Various
Steroids through PDMS[9]

Steroid	Ratio of diffusion rate to that of cortisol[a]
19-Norprogesterone	224
Progesterone	78.2
Testosterone	53.0
Megestrol acetate	39.5
Norethindrone	12.2
Estradiol	10.2
Mestranol	7.2
Corticosterone	3.5
Cortisol	1.0

a.   The diffusion rate of cortisol was
6 $\mu g/(100\ mm^2)(0.1\ mm)(day)$.

Our analysis of these data showed that structural
and chemical features of the steroids did indeed influence the rates of diffusion.

Effects of Structures of the Drugs

The steroidal drugs used for contraception have
obvious similarities in gross structure and differ
primarily in their A-ring functionality and the substituents at the C-10 and C-17 positions. For example,

progesterone   mestranol

A few general statements can be made with regard to
the steric requirements of these steroidal hormones.
(1) The approximate molecular dimensions of the steroidal
ring system including the C-18 and C-19 methyl groups are
5.2 x 7.2 x 17 Å; thus these molecules have a minimum
cross-sectional area of about 36 Å^2.   (2) The approximate
molecular dimensions of the steroidal ring system without
angular C-18 and C-19 methyl groups are 3 x 7.2 x 17 Å;
hence these molecules have a minimum cross-sectional area
of about 22 Å^2.   (3) The molecular dimensions of the
estrogenic steroidal ring system where the A-ring is aromatic (as in mestranol) are approximately 4 x 8.5 x 20 Å;
hence these molecules have a minimum cross-sectional area
of about 34 Å^2.   (4) The presence of two large substituents at the 17-position on the D-ring increases the
minimum cross-sectional area of the molecules significantly since one of the substituents must assume a quasi-
axial conformation.   (5) Some of the steroidal hormones
have highly polar groups in the 3- and 17-positions.   The
degree of polarity of these substituents will influence
the equilibrium solubility of the steroid in the polymer
and the partition coefficient between the steroid in the
polymer and in the solution into which it diffuses.

A brief discussion of the method used in analyzing
Kincl's data and of some of the conclusions reached will
aid in showing the effects of structural features of
steroids on their diffusion rates.

Table II shows the average diffusion rates and the
relative diffusion rates with respect to 19-norprogester-
one of various steroids through a PDMS membrane.   The
differences in structure of the various steroids in
Table II are variations in the A-ring, the C-19 methyl,
or the substituents at the C-17 position of the D-ring.
Since each of the steroids has at least one structural
feature in common with 19-norprogesterone or with
another steroid related to 19-norprogesterone, the
magnitude of the effect of each structural change can
be calculated relative to the rate of diffusion of
19-norprogesterone through PDMS.   These effects of
structural change can be expressed as a "relative diffusivity factor:, which is the ratio of diffusion rates
of two steroids differing in one structural feature.
The calculated "relative diffusivity factors" for structural changes in the steroids are shown in Table III.

Inspection of the structural changes and their effects on diffusion rate shown in Table III allows the

Table II. Diffusion Rates of Various Steroids through
           a Polydimethylsiloxane Membrane

	Average diffusion rate[a]	Relative diffusion rate[b]
19-norprogesterone	1353	1
progesterone	469	0.35
testosterone	317	0.23
norethindrone	73	0.054
estradiol	61	0.045
mestranol	43	0.032

a. Diffusion rate $\mu g/(100 \text{ mm}^2)(0.1 \text{ mm})(\text{day})$.
b. Relative to 19-norprogesterone.

Table III. Effect of Structural Changes on the Rate of Diffusion of Steroids through Polydimethylsiloxane Membranes

<table>
<tr><th colspan="2">Structural change</th><th>Relative diffusivity factor</th></tr>
<tr><td>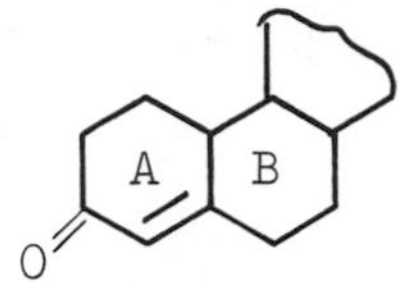
</td><td>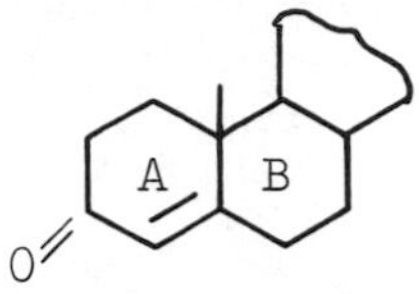
</td><td>0.35</td></tr>
<tr><td>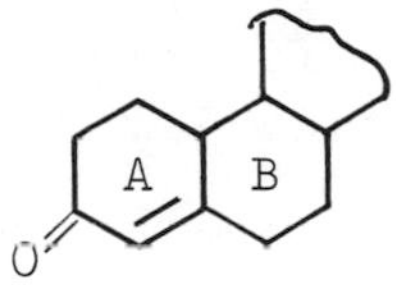
</td><td>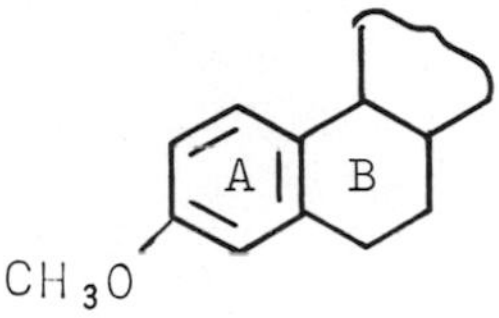
</td><td>0.59</td></tr>
<tr><td>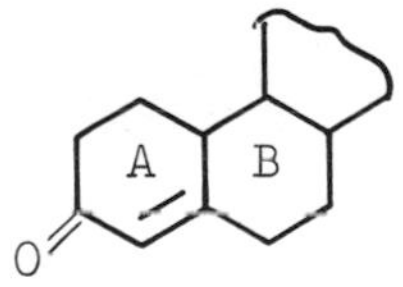
</td><td>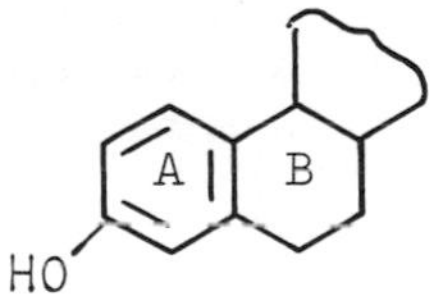
</td><td>0.066</td></tr>
<tr><td>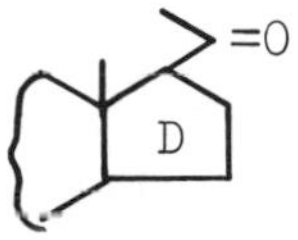
</td><td>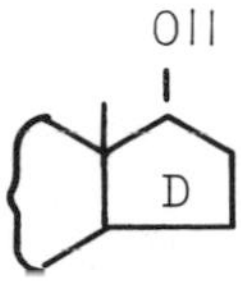
</td><td>0.68</td></tr>
<tr><td>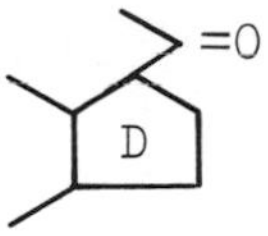
</td><td>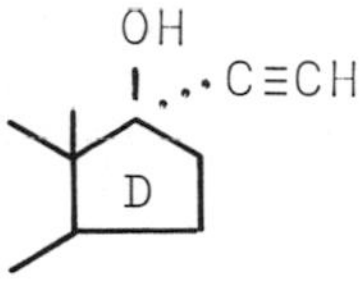
</td><td>0.054</td></tr>
<tr><td>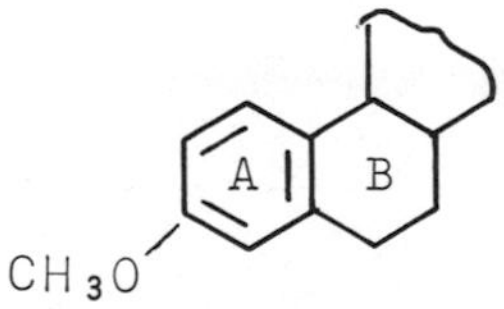
</td><td>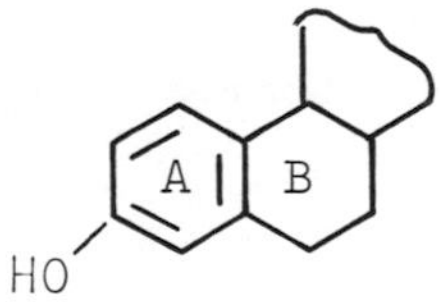
</td><td>0.12</td></tr>
<tr><td>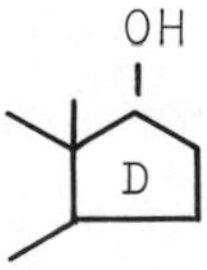
</td><td>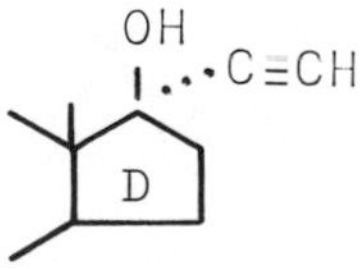
</td><td>0.080</td></tr>
</table>

following conclusions to be drawn. (1) The addition of
a C-19 angular methyl substituent increases the steric
requirement of the molecule and alters the relative diffusivity through PDMS by 0.35 (i.e., the diffusion rate
of the steroid with an angular C-19 methyl group is 0.35
times that of a steroid without the C-19 methyl group).
(2) Changing the A-ring from alicylic 3-keto to aromatic
3-methoxy increases the steric requirement slightly and
alters the relative diffusivity through PDMS by 0.59.
(3) Changing the 3-substituent on an aromatic A-ring
from methoxy to hydroxy does not significantly alter the
steric requirement of the molecule; however, a large
change (a factor of 0.12) in the relative diffusivity
through PDMS occurs probably due to the lower solubility
of the more highly polar molecule in the silicone. (4)
Changing the methylketo group at the C-17 position of
the D-ring to hydroxy likewise does not significantly
alter the steric requirement of the molecule, but a
small change (0.68) in the relative diffusivity through
PDMS occurs due to increased polarity causing decreased
solubility. (5) Changing the C-17 position of the D-
ring by adding an ethynyl group, which has a large
steric requirement due to its rigidity, to a 17-hydroxy
D-ring group alters the relative diffusivity of the
steroid through PDMS significantly (0.080). Such relationships between structure and diffusion rates could
be of great value to designers of drug-release systems
because the relationships could permit the prediction
of the diffusion rates of other similar drugs through a
given type of membrane without substantial experimental
effort. For example, on the basis of Kincl's reported
value of 317 $\mu g/(100 \text{ mm}^2)(0.1 \text{ mm})(\text{day})$ for the diffusion
rate of testosterone through PDMS and with the data in
Table III for the effect of removing an angular methyl
group from the 19-position on the steroid ring, the diffusion rate of 19-nortestosterone through PDMS should
be about 317/0.35 or 905 $\mu g/(100 \text{ mm}^2)(0.1 \text{ mm})(\text{day})$. The
relationships between changes in the structure of
steroids and changes in the basic diffusional factors,
C_m, D, and K would be of much greater predictive value.

We therefore selected, for our initial studies, the
following series of steroids in which each steroid dif-
fers from the one above it in the series by only one
structural feature. We determined C_m, D, and K for each
steroid through PDMS.

norprogesterone

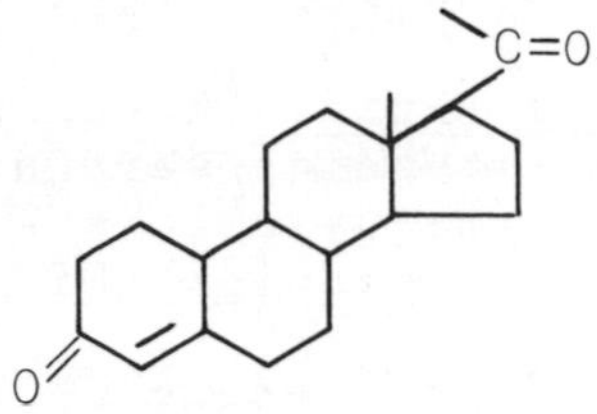

progesterone

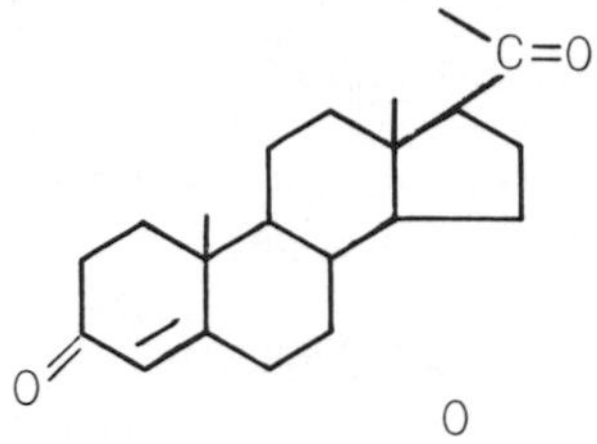

androstenedione

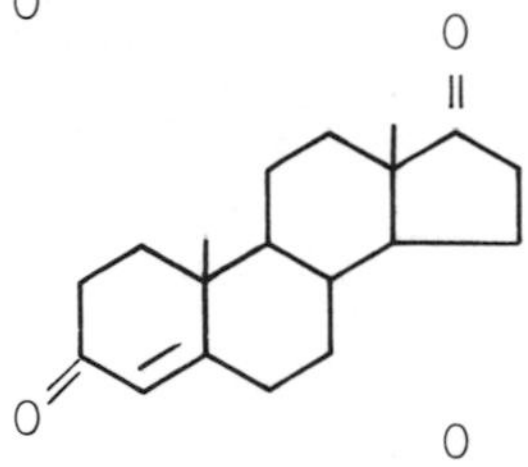

estrone

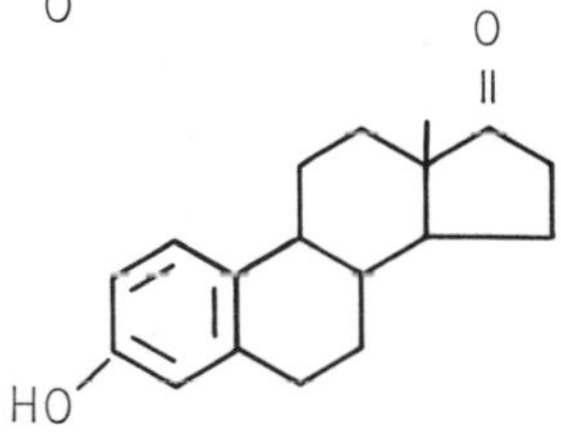

IV.   EXPERIMENTAL

Materials

Membranes.   The PDMS used to make membranes for these studies was the MDX4-4092 fluid and catalyst system of the Dow Corning Corporation, Midland, Michigan (Lot E914-32).   As received, MDX4-4092 is a fluid comprising hydroxy-terminated dimethylsiloxane polymer and a cross-linking agent.   A separate catalyst system is furnished. To prepare membranes, catalyst was added to a weighed amount of MDX4-4092 and the catalyzed liquid was intro-duced into a 3 x 3-in. spin-casting cup.   The fluid polymer was spread into a 0.05-cm film by the centri-fugal force provided by the spin caster, and vulcaniza-tion took place at room temperature to form the membrane.

The average chain length of the polymer determined
by gel permeation chromatography was 3000 Å.

Suspending fluid. The fluids studied as suspending
media for the steroids were deionized water and a polytrifluoropropylmethylsiloxane designated as FS1265 fluid
(Dow Corning Corporation, Midland, Michigan).

Steroids. The progesterone used in these studies
was obtained from the Sigma Chemical Company, St. Louis,
Missouri. The 19-norprogesterone was a gift from Syntex
Research, Palo Alto, California; the androst-4-ene-3,17-
dione was a gift from Searle Laboratories, Chicago,
Illinois; and the estrone was a gift from The Upjohn
Company, Kalamazoo, Michigan. Each steroid was mixed
with its tritium-labeled counterpart obtained from New
England Nuclear, Boston, Massachusetts to provide the
desired specific activity.

Experimental Procedures

Solubilities. A satisfactory procedure for determining the equilibrium solubilities of steroids in PDMS must
ensure no contamination of the PDMS sample by adhering or
adsorbed steroid. To avoid contamination catalyzed fluid
PDMS was drawn into a small poly(vinyl chloride) (PVC)
tube from which plasticizer had been extracted. The PDMS
was allowed to crosslink and solidify in the PVC tube.
After storing these tubes overnight to ensure completion
of the crosslinking reaction, the tubes of PDMS encased
in PVC were cut into 4-mm lengths. Many of these samples
were equilibrated with powdered tritium-labeled steroid
(specific activity = 2.5 µC/mg) at 37°C in vials shaken
in a water bath.

After seven days samples were removed. The encased
samples were rinsed three times by immersing them in
methyl alcohol for 2 seconds. The sample was blotted
dry, and the PVC tube was slit axially and removed from
the PDMS core. Since the rinsing procedure could have
extracted some steroid from the unprotected ends of the
PDMS, a 0.5-mm section was sliced from each end of the
sample and discarded.

These samples were weighed and then extracted with
methylene chloride in micro-Soxhlet extractors. The
solvent was evaporated to dryness and the residues were

taken up in 15 ml of scintillation counting fluid.* Counts of radioactivity were made in a Packard Tri-Carb scintillation spectrophotometer. The concentrations of steroid in the polymer were calculated from the weights and specific gravities of the polymers, and the counts and specific activities of the steroids.

The withdrawal of samples and subsequent processing of samples to obtain counts of radioactivity were repeated at one-week intervals until equilibrium was assured.

Solubilities of steroids in water were determined by equilibrating a number of vials containing excess solid steroid in water by shaking the vials at 37°C in a water bath. Vials containing solution were removed from the bath at 1-day intervals, and centrifuged to separate the solids. (Filtration through 0.22-micron Millipore filters proved unacceptable due to sorption of steroids by the cellulose acetate filters.) A 1-ml sample of the clear supernatant solution was withdrawn with a pipette, and mixed with 14 ml of aqueous scintillation counting fluid.** Counts of radioactivity were made, and the concentration of steroid was calculated from the counts and specific activities.

With the exception of estrone, the solubilities of steroids in FS1265 were determined by the method used for solutions in water. Estrone and FS1265 had similar specific gravities so that separation of solids by centrifugation was difficult. For estrone the solid steroid was placed in small bags fabricated from Nuclepore® membranes. The bags were sealed and placed in vials containing FS1265, and the contents were equilibrated at 37°C by shaking the vials in a water bath. This method proved satisfactory, but long times for equilibration (up to 30 days) were necessary.

---

*Made by mixing 1 gal of toluene with 160 ml of Liquiflor® (trademark registered by New England Nuclear, Boston, Massachusetts).

**Made by mixing 240 g of naphthalene, 330 ml of toluene, 330 ml of ethoxyethanol, 2340 ml of p-dioxane, and 25 ml of Omnifluor® (trademark registered by New England Nuclear, Boston, Massachusetts).

®Trademark registered by the Nuclepore Division of The General Electric Company.

   Partition coefficients. Partition coefficients were
calculated from the separately determined equilibrium
solubilities in polymer and in fluids (water and FS1265).
They were also determined by equilibration of polymer in
solutions by the method described below.

   Saturated solutions of steroids in water and in
FS1265 were prepared by the method described previously.
After separation of the solids, 5-ml samples of the clear
solutions were placed in test tubes, to which preweighed
small samples of membranes were added. The tubes were
equilibrated by shaking them at 37°C in a water bath. At
timed intervals membrane samples were withdrawn from the
solutions, wiped with a Kim-wipe moistened with methyl
alcohol, blotted dry, and weighed.

   These samples were extracted with methylene chloride
in micro-Soxhlet extractors. The solvent was evaporated
to dryness, and the residues were taken up in 15 ml of
scintillation counting fluid (toluene and Liquifluor).
Counts of radioactivity were made, and the concentrations
of steroids in the polymer were calculated.

   At each withdrawal of a membrane sample a 1-ml sample
of the fluid, which was no longer saturated, was also
withdrawn. These samples were taken up in an appropriate
scintillation counting fluid (the aqueous fluid for
aqueous samples; toluene and Liquifluor for FS1265*), and
counts of radioactivity were made. The concentrations of
steroids in the fluids were calculated from the counts
and specific activities. Values of partition coefficients were calculated from the concentrations of
steroids in the polymer and in the fluids. The procedure was repeated at longer time intervals to determine when equilibration had occurred.

   Diffusion coefficients. A sketch of the diffusion
cell is shown in Figure 2. One of the half-cells has a
reservoir for steroids, which may be present either as
dry powders or as pastes of particles suspended in a
fluid. The other half-cell has a channel provided with
an inlet and outlet tube to permit the introduction and
withdrawal of solution that circulates through that half
of the cell. The solution is circulated at a high rate
(about 400 ml/min) through this half of the cell to reduce the thickness of the diffusional boundary layers

---

*One milliliter of Soluene® (a solubilizing agent ob-
tained from the Packard Instrument Company, Downers
Grove, Illinois) had to be added to the FS1265 to enhance its solubility in the toluene counting fluid.

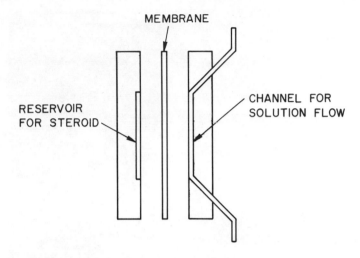

Figure 2.   Sketch of Diffusion Cell

adjacent to the membrane. No solution flows through the
steroid reservoir, but with solids or pastes the diffusional boundary layer is very thin because the solid
particles of steroid are held against the membrane. The
combined thickness of the two boundary layers was calculated to be 14 to 16 microns, which was also the calculated thickness of the combined layers obtained by
Roseman[21] in a different type of diffusion cell.

The complete cell is assembled by placing the
steroid-reservoir half-cell flat, introducing the
steroid as either a dry powder or a paste, smoothing
the membrane onto the surface of the half-cell, placing
the other half-cell on top of the membrane, and clamp-
ing the half-cells together.

The assembled diffusion cell is mounted in a circulation loop as shown in the sketch in Figure 3 and in
the photograph in Figure 4. In addition to the diffusion
cell the circulation loop is provided with a flowmeter,
a thermometer with a temperature sensor set at 37°C, a
filling funnel, a section heated by heating tapes, a
drain tube, and a specially made mercury-seal pump.
Originally, a peristaltic pump was used to circulate
the solution, but was found to be unsuitable because the
poly(vinyl chloride) tubing in the peristaltic pump
adsorbed much of the steroids transferred through the
membrane. Therefore, the mercury-seal pump was installed.

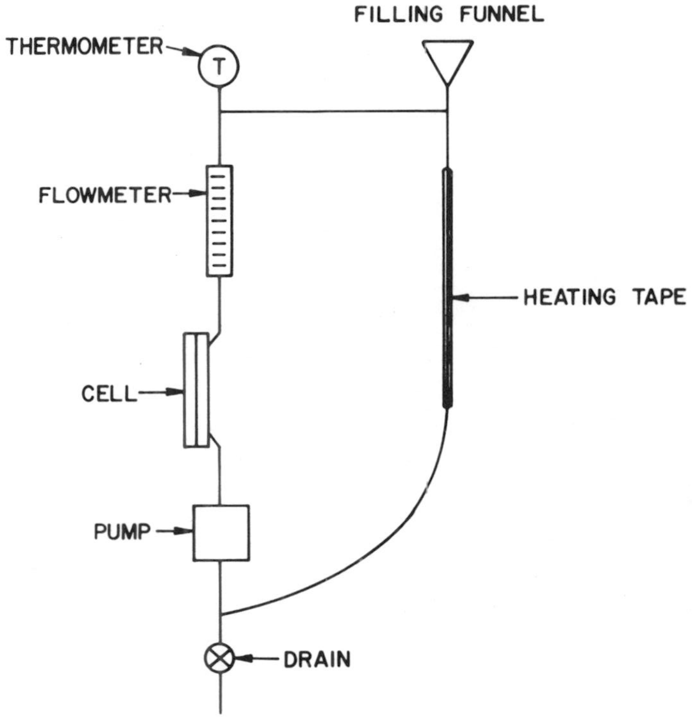

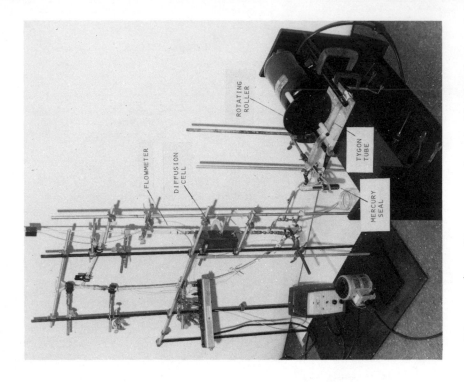

Figure 4. Photograph of diffusion apparatus.

Figure 3. Sketch of diffusion apparatus showing circulation loop.

The mercury-seal pump shown in Figure 4 consists of a Tygon tube filled with water and connected to a mercury seal made from a vapor trap used with vacuum pumps. A roller mounted eccentrically on a disk rotated by a con-trollable-speed motor compresses the Tygon tubing during each rotation of the disk. The compression forces water into the mercury-seal device and imparts a reciprocating motion to the mercury. Each complete pulse of the mer-cury column first pulls solution from the circulation loop through a bottom check valve, and then forces that amount of solution through a top check valve back into the circulating loop.

For best operation, the speed of the pump was ad-justed to the natural resonant frequency of the mercury column, which was 94 pulses per minute. At this speed the pump delivered 400 ml/min, which resulted in an average velocity through the flow channel in the dif-fusion cell of 35 cm/sec.

The temperature of the solution in the circulating loop was controlled to 37±0.2°C by a temperature sensor set at 37°C on the extended-scale thermometer in the loop. This temperature sensor actuated a Matheson Lab-stat that turned the electrical current to the heating tapes on or off.

V.   RESULTS AND DISCUSSION

Values of solubilities, partition coefficients, and diffusion coefficients were determined for all four steroids.

Solubilities

Solubilities measured at 37°C of the four steroids in PDMS, FS1265 (a potential suspending fluid), and water are given in Table IV. Six to twenty-two measure-ments of the solubility of each steroid were made. The mean values of solubilities, the standard deviation of the mean value (i.e., standard error), and the 95%-confidence range are given in Table IV. The mean value for the solubility of progesterone of 12.6 µg/ml cor-responds closely with two values given in the literature (11 µg/ml,[21] and 12.6 µg/ml[22]), but does not compare well with a third value given in the literature (27 µg/ml[10]).

Table IV. Solubilities of Selected Steroids in Polymers and Fluids at 37°C

Equilibrium solubility, μg/ml
(number of measurements in parentheses)

Steroid	In PDMS[a]			In FS1265[d]			In water		
	Mean value	$s_{\bar{x}}$[b]	Range[c]	Mean value	$s_{\bar{x}}$[b]	Range[c]	Mean value	$s_{\bar{x}}$[b]	Range[c]
Norprogesterone	631 (8)	28	575 to 687	2306 (11)	133	2041 to 2571	36.1 (28)	1.3	33.5 to 38.7
Progesterone	763 (19)	16	731 to 795	2050 (10)	28	1994 to 2106	12.6 (36)	0.2	12.2 to 13.0
Androstenedione	365 (19)	14	337 to 393	1765 (11)	25	1715 to 1815	48.7 (47)	1.1	46.5 to 50.9
Estrone	324 (9)	32	260 to 388	33 (6)	2	29 to 37	3.2 (40)	0.03	3.1 to 3.3

a. Crosslinked polydimethylsiloxane. MDX4-4092 polymer system from the Dow Corning Corporation.
b. $s_{\bar{x}}$ = standard deviation of the mean value, sometimes termed the standard error.
c. Range = mean value $\pm 2\ s_{\bar{x}}$; the 95%-confidence range.
d. Polytrifluoropropylmethylsiloxane fluid. No. FS1265 fluid from the Dow Corning Corporation.

The same reference[10] gave for the solubility of norprogesterone in water at 37°C a value of 12 µg/ml, which
does not correspond closely with the value of 36.1 µg/ml
given in Table IV. No data on the solubilities of
estrone or androstenedione were found in the literature.
However, estrogenic steroids other than estrone for
which data were found in the literature also had very
low solubilities in water (estradiol, 5 µg/ml, and
mestranol, 1.5 µg/ml[10]).

Partition Coefficients

Mean values of partition coefficients, K, that were
determined from solubilities in the polymer and in water
(measured separately and given in Table IV) are listed
in Table V as "calculated" values. Partition coefficients determined by equilibration of polymer samples in
solutions of the steroids in water are listed also in
Table V as "nonsaturated" values. The concentrations of
the steroids in water for the calculated values or at
the final value of concentration reached in the equilibration tests are given in parentheses in Table V. Similar data for the partition coefficients of steroids
between PDMS and FS1265 are given in Table VI.

In the absence of interfering phenomena the calculated values and the nonsaturated values of K should be
the same. For progesterone and androstenedione the
values of K in Table V, which were calculated from the
solubilities at saturation, are almost identical with
those determined below saturation. For norprogesterone
the two values of K are similar. However, for estrone
the value of K below saturation is much lower than that
calculated for saturation. The values of K given in
Table VI for the partitioning of steroids between FS1265
and PDMS are all lower below saturation than at saturation.

The possible causes of the lack of correspondence
between the values of K determined by the two methods
are: (a) equilibrium might not have been attained in
determining either K or C, or both; (b) some of the
fluid used in determining the equilibrium values of K
might have permeated the PDMS and altered the partitioning; and (c) the steroids could be associated in either
the fluid or the polymer phase.

The attainment of equilibrium in the determination
of both C and K was checked by taking samples after

Table V. Partition Coefficients for Steroids
between Water and Polydimethylsiloxane

| Steroid | Partition coefficient | | | | | |
| | Calculated value | | | Nonsaturated value | | |
	Mean value	$s\bar{x}$ [a]	Range [b]	Mean value	$s\bar{x}$ [a]	Range [b]
Norprogesterone	17.5	0.9	15.7 to 19.3 µg/ml	22.4	0.91	20.6 to 24.2 µg/ml
	(sat'd concn = 36.1 µg/ml)			(at a concn of 11.8 µg/ml)		
Progesterone	60.5	3.00	54.5 to 66.5 µg/ml	59.4	2.1	55.2 to 63.6 µg/ml
	(sat'd concn = 12.6 µg/ml)			(at a concn of 4.7 µg/ml)		
Androstenedione	7.5	1.15	5.2 to 9.8 µg/ml	7.4	0.07	7.3 to 7.5 µg/ml
	(sat'd concn = 48.7 µg/ml)			(at a concn of 13.3 µg/ml)		
Estrone	102	9.0	84 to 120 µg/ml	8.0	0.77	6.5 to 9.5 µg/ml
	(sat'd concn = 3.1 µg/ml)			(at a concn of 2.4 µg/ml)		

a. $s\bar{x}$ = standard deviation of the mean value.
b. Range = mean value ±2 $s\bar{x}$, is the 95%-confidence range.

Table VI. Partition Coefficients for Steroids between FS1265[a] and Polydimethylsiloxane

| | Partition coefficient | | | | | |
| | Calculated value | | | Nonsaturated value | | |
Steroid	Mean value	$s_{\bar{x}}$ [b]	Range [c]	Mean value	$s_{\bar{x}}$ [b]	Range [c]
Norprogesterone	0.24	0.011	0.22 to 0.26 (at a concn of 2306 µg/ml)	0.108	0.005	0.098 to 0.118 (at a concn of 1647 µg/ml)
Progesterone	0.47	0.05	0.51 to 0.61 (at a concn of 1613 µg/ml)	0.127	0.005	0.117 to 0.137 (at a concn of 1115 µg/ml)
Androstenedione	0.17	0.008	0.15 to 0.19 (at a concn of 1765 µg/ml)	0.101	0.008	0.085 to 0.117 (at a concn of 1310 µg/ml)
Estrone	6.8	1.0	4.8 to 8.8 (at a concn of 33 µg/ml)	1.65	0.14	1.37 to 1.93 (at a concn of 23 µg/ml)

a. Polytrifluoropropylmethylsiloxane fluid from the Dow Corning Corporation.
b. Standard deviation of the mean value.
c. Range = mean value ± 2 $s_{\bar{x}}$, is the 95%-confidence range.

successive elapsed times until the same values (of C or
K) were obtained at two or more times. It seems probable that equilibrium was achieved.

Absorption of fluid by the membrane, with consequent
alteration of partition coefficients, is not clearly evident. If absorption of water had occurred, the values
of K for progesterone and androstenedione below saturation should have been lower, and if absorption of FS1265
had occurred, the values of K below saturation should
have been higher than the calculated values of K. Experiments of Most[23] showed that permeation of a polymer
by a substance in which a drug is more soluble than it
is in the polymer resulted in a higher solubility of the
drug in the polymer-permeant combination than in the
polymer alone.

Because the experimental evidence does not correspond
to the findings of Most,[23] it would seem that fluid permeation of the polymer is not responsible for the observed differences in the values of K.

A third hypothesized cause of the differences is
that the steroids are associated in either the fluid or
the polymer phase. We believe this is the most probable
reason for the lack of correspondence of the values of
K. If the steroids were associated in the fluid, the
expression for the partition coefficient can be written
as:

$$K = \frac{C_{polymer}}{C_{fluid}(1 - \beta)}$$

where: K = partition coefficient

$C_{polymer}$ = concentration of steroid in
                polymer (assumed to be
                nonassociated)

C_{fluid} = concentration of steroid in
              fluid (assumed to be
              associated)

β = degree of association

The steroids could be associated in both fluid and
polymer phases, but to different degrees, and a similar
expression could be developed to contain a term, β_p, for
degree of association in the polymer, and term, β_f, for
degree of association in the fluid phase.

Experiments are needed to test the validity of this hypothesis that association is the cause of the differences in measured solubilities in the polymer and those predicted by the KC products.

Diffusion Coefficients

The diffusion coefficients of the four steroids in PDMS as calculated by the time-lag method are given in Table VII. Values of the standard deviation of the mean and the 95%-confidence range are also given.

In general, the variations of the diffusion coefficients shown in Table VII appear to be related to structure approximately as expected. The presence of the 19-methyl group in progesterone, compared with its absence in norprogesterone, reduced the diffusion coefficient (a conductance term) from 18.5×10^{-7} cm^2 sec^{-1} to 6.4×10^{-7} cm^2 sec^{-1}. The replacement of the rather bulky keto-group at the 17-position in progesterone with the less bulky double-bond oxygen substituent in androstenedione resulted in an increase in D to 14.8×10^{-7} cm^2 sec^{-1}.

The difference between D for androstenedione and that for estrone probably reflects changes in chemical nature as well as in strucutre. Estrone lacks the 19-methyl group of androstenedione. In view of the increase in D from the absence of a 19-methyl group (compare progesterone and norprogesterone), the value of D for estrone should be larger than that for androstenedione, if structural changes alone affected D. Instead, the value of D for estrone in considerably smaller (2.4×10^{-7} cm^2 sec^{-1} compared with 14.8×10^{-7} cm^2 sec^{-1}). The most probable change other than the structural change that affects D for this pair of steroids is the change in the chemical nature of the A-ring. The A-ring of androstenedione is an alicyclic unsaturated ketone, whereas the A-ring of estrone is an aromatic phenol. Two molecules of estrone could be hydrogen-bonded together within the membrane to form a bulky complex that would be severely restricted in its movement. There also could be much stronger chemical interactions between the A-ring of estrone and the siloxane polymer segments than between the alicyclic A-ring of androstenedione and the segments.

Table VII. Diffusion Coefficients of
Steroids in PDMS

Steroid	Structures	Diffusion coefficient, cm^2/sec		
		Mean value	$s_{\bar{x}}$ [a]	Range x (10^7) [b]
Norprogesterone		18.5 x 10^{-7}	2.5	13.5 to 23.5
Progesterone		6.4 x 10^{-7}	0.3	5.8 to 7.0
Androstenedione		14.8 x 10^{-7}	1.2	12.4 to 17.4
Estrone		2.4 x 10^{-7}	0.3	1.8 to 3.0

a. $s_{\bar{x}}$ = Standard deviation of the mean value, some-
    times termed the standard error.

b. Range = Mean value ±2 $s_{\bar{x}}$. There is 95% confidence
    that the mean value is in this range.

ACKNOWLEDGMENT

     The authors wish to acknowledge the support of the
National Institutes of Health under Contract NIH-NICHD-
72-2768 with the National Institutes of Health, Department of Health, Education, and Welfare. We would also
like to acknowledge the valuable contributions to the
research of Mrs. Gloria Elston, Assistant Biologist,
Mrs. Sarah Perkins, Laboratory Helper, and Mr. Ronnie
Bayless, Research Technician. We are grateful for the
gifts of steroids by Searle Laboratories, Syntex
Research, and The Upjohn Company.

REFERENCES

1. P. J. Dziuk and B. Cook, Endocrinology, 78, 208
    (1966).

2. J. Folkman and D. Long, Ann. N. Y. Acad. Sci., 111,
    857 (1964).

3. J. Folkman and D. Long, Science, 154, 148 (1966).

4. P. Bass, R. Purdon, and J. Riley, Nature, 208,
    591 (1965).

5. K. G. Powers, J. Parasitology, 51 (Sec. 2), 53
    (1965).

6. S. J. Segal, in "Future Prospects in Contraception",
    Proc. of The Fifth World Congress on Fertility and
    Sterility, Stockholm, June 1966, Int'l Congr. Ser.,
    113, 1028 (1967).

7. E. Garrett and P. Chemburkar, (a) J. Pharm. Sci.,
    57, 944 (1968); (b) J. Pharm. Sci., 57, 949 (1968).

8. E. Garrett and P. Chemburkar, J. Pharm. Sci., 57,
    140 (1968).

9. F. Kincl, G. Benagiano, and I. Angee, Steroids, 11,
    673 (1968).

10. K. Sundaram and F. Kincl, Steroids, 12, 517 (1968).

11. P. Kratochvil, G. Benagiano, and F. Kincl, Steroids,
    15, 505 (1970).

12. S. Friedman, S. Koide, and F. Kincl, Steroids, 15,
     679 (1970).

13. H. A. Daynes, Proc. Roy. Soc. London, A97, 286
     (1920).

14. R. M. Barrer, Trans. Farad. Soc., 35, 628 (1939).

15. A. Lifchez and A. Scommegna, Fertil. and Steril.,
     21, 426 (1970).

16. D. Mishell, M. Talas, A. Parlow, and D. Moyer,
     Amer. J. Obstet. and Gynec., 107, 100 (1970).

17. D. Mishell and M. Lumkin, Fertil. and Steril.,
     21, 99 (1970).

18. T. Roseman and W. I. Higuchi, J. Pharm. Sci., 59,
     353 (1970).

19. H. Croxatto, S. Diaz, R. Vera, M. Etchart, and
     P. Atria, Amer. J. Obstet. and Gynec., 104, 1135
     (1969).

20. H. Tatum, E. Coutinho, J. A. Filho, and A. Sant'Anna,
     Amer. J. Obstet. and Gynec., 105, 1139 (1969).

21. T. J. Roseman, J. Pharm. Sci., 61, 46 (1972).

22. F. Bischoff and H. Pilhorn, J. Biol. Chem., 174,
     663 (1948).

23. C. F. Most, J. Biomed. Mater. Res., 6, 3 (1972).

DEVELOPMENT OF A DELIVERY SYSTEM FOR PROSTAGLANDINS

E. S. Nuwayser and D. L. Williams

Abcor, Inc., 341 Vassar Street

Cambridge, Massachusetts   02139

I.   INTRODUCTION

Much of the research on implantable capsules for contraception involves diffusion of steroids through polydimethylsiloxane (PDMS). The capsules have been implanted intramuscularly, subcutaneously or into adipose tissue. They have been tested also as intra-uterine devices or vaginal rings.

Among the earlier studies in this field, Doyle and Clewe[1] employed a capsule prepared by admixing meleng-estrol acetate with PDMS and reported contraceptive effect by intrauterine implantation in rats and rabbits. A similar capsule containing progesterone was tested in women by Mishell and Lumkin[2] with demonstrated success. The studies of Kincl et al.[3-6] were based on the use of a small hollow tube made of PDMS, with various steroids encapsulated in the lumen. Work by Scommegna et al.[7-9] and Dziuk and Cook[10] was based on the hollow-tube cap-sule approach as well. Very recent work by Croxatto et al.[11] demonstrated the effectiveness of the method for contraception in women over 9-12 month periods. The effect of co-permeant enhancement of benzocaine trans-mission through silicone rubber was studied by Most.[12] The use of silicone discs for the sustained release of chloroquin diphosphate was studied by Fu et al.[13] and the controlled release of testosterone using cylinders of the same polymer was reported by Shippy et al.[14]

From the above discussion, it is evident that the
use of capsules for the controlled delivery of biologically active agents will offer significant advantages
over oral or intravenous administration. This was established in studies of capsules for the delivery of
steroid hormones. First, apparently much lower dosages
can be effectively administered with the implanted capsule in contrast to oral usage and subcutaneous injection.[5]   Second, drug delivery at the site (uterus or
cervix) can result in fewer detrimental side effects.[8]
Third, when the hollow-tube approach is taken, a constant
rate of release is experienced.[3,7]

The objective of this work was to develop methods
for the controlled release of prostaglandin $PGF_{2\alpha}$
which is based on its transport properties through semi-
permeable membranes. In such membranes, the rate of
mass transport is controlled by membrane permeation.
The release of the drug from a membrane capsule is directly proportional to the membrane surface area and
inversely proportional to its thickness. The approach
is based on the development of implantable capillary
membrane microcapsules which contain the desired prostaglandin and deliver it at a prescribed rate. The microcapsule is designed for implantation in the lower uterus,
between the fetal membrane and the uterine wall. The
small diameter of the microcapsule would facilitate its
insertion through the cervical os and its placement in
the target area.

Early in the program target dose rates for the PGE_2
microcapsules were formulated after consultation with
Professor Sultan M. Karim of Makerere University Medical
School in Kampala, Uganda. Two dose rates were developed,
one for use in early pregnancy and the other for late
(second trimester) pregnancy (Table I). Most of our
studies were conducted with the latter. This rate comprises an initial high dose component (2.5 mg per hour
for 2 hours) and a constant longer term component (1.0
mg per hr for next 10 hours). The function of the
initial component is to stimulate contractions of the
uterine wall smooth muscle, whereas the longer term
component will maintain this state for a period during which abortion is expected to occur. Recent
clinical reports[15] with extra-amniotic infusion of PG
indicate that the dose may have to be increased and the
period extended as long as 28-30 hours. The second
trimester target dose rate schedules established for
PGE_2 were used for the development of the $PGF_{2\alpha}$ capillary microcapsule.

Table I.   Target Prostaglandin E$_2$
Release Rates

PREGNANCY TIME		INITIAL INCREMENT	CONSTANT RELEASE	TOTAL
EARLY	RATE	0.05 MG/HR x 1 HR	0.05 MG/HR x 12 HR	0.65 MG
	TOTAL	0.05 MG	0.60 MG	0.65 MG
	PER CENT	8%	92%	100%
LATE	RATE	1.5 MG/HR x 2 HR	1.0 MG/HR x 12 HR	15 MG
	TOTAL	3.0 MG	12 MG	15 MG
	PER CENT	20%	80%	100%

II.   PROPERTIES OF PROSTAGLANDINS

Prostaglandins are derivatives of "prostanoic acid",
a trivial name proposed by Bergstrom et al.[16] to describe
the hypothetical lipid molecule upon which the name of
these biologically active compounds was based.   The molecule is a cyclic, C$_{20}$ oxygenated fatty acid.   Its configuration is shown in Figure 1.   Natural prostaglandins
are produced from the corresponding polyunsaturated fatty
acids by a microsomal synthetase system.   The work with
prostaglandins (PG) for the induction of therapeutic
abortion was done with PGE$_1$ and PGF$_{2\alpha}$, whose structures
are also shown in Figure 1.   Their mode of action depends
on their ability to stimulate uterine smooth muscle.
Most of our studies were conducted with PGF$_{2\alpha}$ and some
with PGE$_1$.

The administration of prostaglandins is further com-
plicated as a result of rapid deactivation in the body.
Naturally released prostaglandins normally have a local
or regional effect without traversing normal routes of
blood circulation.   There are many examples of prostaglandins detected in the venous effluent from an organ.
However the liver deactivates up to 90% of the PGE$_1$,
PGE$_2$, or PGF$_{2\alpha}$ which passes through it.   The lungs have
a similar function and deactivate up to 95% of these
prostaglandins with one pass through the pulmonary circulation.[17]   The action of the lungs is primarily due to
the enzyme prostaglandin 15-dehydrogenase.   Hence this
position is normally protected by substitution in the
preparation of longer lasting analogues.

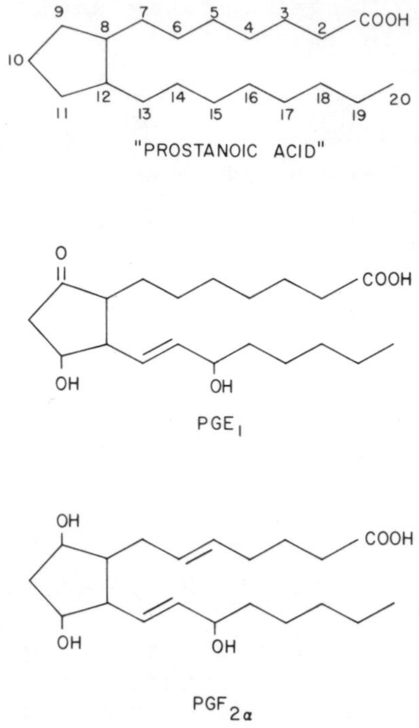

Figure 1. Structure of Prostaglandins

Although much effort has been placed on preparing prostaglandin analogues which will not be as readily deactivated, the most direct approach is to use a slow-release implanted capsule filled with prostaglandin. Longer acting analogues may be also encapsulated to further increase their effectiveness. The use of analogues which are activated by hydrolysis necessitates higher initial concentrations and will not have the advantage of the localized effect of an implanted capsule.

The solubility of $PGF_{2\alpha}$ THAM salt [tris(hydroxymethyl)aminomethane] has been found to be very great. However, at greater than a one-to-one concentration, the solutions are tacky. The solubility of the free acid PGE_1 in water was found to be 1.4 mg/ml. This value was determined by saturating a solution with the radioactively tagged prostaglandin and measuring the radioactivity of the supernate.

Capillary Diffusion

Most of the literature on drug release uses equations based on planar diffusion. Our systems are small capillaries in which radial diffusion occurs. The fundamental equation for radial diffusion is given by Crank:[18]

$$Q_t = \frac{2\pi Dt(C_2 - C_1)}{\ln \frac{r_o}{r_i}} \qquad (1)$$

where

Q_t = quantity released per unit length of capillary in time t

D = diffusion coefficient in cm^2/sec

C_1 = concentration of drug outside the capsule

C_2 = concentration of drug inside the capsule

r_i = inside radius, ID/2

r_o = outside radius, OD/2

For purposes of calculation, we will assume that $C_1 = 0$ or $C_2 \gg C_1$. This equation defines the steady state release of prostaglandin, assuming an invariant concentration inside the capillary. This would be true in the presence of solid prostaglandin.

With a solution of prostaglandin, $C_2 = (Q_0 - Q_t)/V$, where Q_0 is the quantity initially in a unit length of fiber, and $V = \pi r_i^2$. Thus, we have a logarithmically decreasing release of prostaglandin. The equation is:

$$Q_t = Q_0 - Q_0 \exp\left[-\frac{2D}{r_i^2 \ln \frac{r_o}{r_i}}\right] t \qquad (2)$$

This equation can be simplified for the analysis of release of 63% $(1 - e^{-1})$ of the material as follows:

$$t_a = \frac{r_i^2 \ln \frac{r_o}{r_i}}{2D} \qquad (3)$$

In the preceding equations, the diffusion coefficient
is an apparent value which includes the partition coefficient between water and the polymer. Thus, the permeability is directly related to the solubility of prostaglandin in the capillary membrane.

In the presence of solid prostaglandin when the polymer and the liquid are both at equilibrium (saturated)
with the solid, the concentration of prostaglandin in the
liquid is constant and is determined by the partition coefficient. However, if this apparent solubility is too
low a considerable resistance to diffusion will be present
in the water or solvent.

With fibers of 10 and 14 mil inside and outside
diameters, respectively, the wall volume may be equal to
the lumen volume. Because of this relatively high wall
volume, the nonsteady state of diffusion into and from
this wall acquires greater importance. Thus, preceding
the quasi-steady state diffusion of the capsule contents
there will be a lag time. In real situations, the induction period before prostaglandin release will also
depend on liquid permeability into the capsule and the
solution rate of dry prostaglandin. Unfortunately, because of the small size of the lumen relative to the
wall, the assumption of a separate non-equilibrium diffusion in the wall may not be applicable. For simplicity, these factors are best determined experimentally.

The diffusion coefficient of the fiber may be determined by one of two methods as follows. The time
(t_a) at which Q_t/Q_o = 63% (i.e., $1 - e^{-1}$) is determined.
At this point the value of D can be found, using Equation (2). Thus:

$$D = \frac{r_i^2 \ln \frac{r_o}{r_i}}{2} \quad \frac{1}{t_a} \tag{4}$$

Alternatively, one may plot log $(1 - Q_t/Q_o)$ vs time using
semilog paper. Thus:

$$D = \frac{r_i^2 \ln \frac{r_o}{r_i}}{2} \quad \frac{2.3 \; \Delta\log (1 - Q_t/Q_o)}{\Delta t} \tag{5}$$

III.   MATERIALS AND METHODS

Materials

Several different materials were melt extruded into
capillary form using a specially designed extruder. The
materials studied were ethylcellulose; cellulose acetate;
cellulose butyrate; silicone rubber; silicone polycarbonate; and nylon. Cellulose acetate and butyrate
capillaries were also modified by removing the plasticizers (phthalates and citrates) and by partially hydro-
lyzing the ester. Other cellulose fiber capillaries were
prepared by dip coating stainless-steel mandrils in polymer solution.

Methods

Radioactive (tritium labeled) and non-radioactive
samples of $PGF_{2\alpha}$ and PGE_1 were obtained courtesy of the
Worcester Foundation for Experimental Biology. PGE_1
was used in place of PGE_2 because of the availability
of radioactive PGE_1. Diffusional properties of these
prostaglandins should almost be identical. The dialysate was analyzed in a scintillation counter.

For diffusion studies the capillary tube was cut
into 10-cm-long sections and filled with prostaglandin
solution. Capillary action was usually enough to fill
the tube. Non-wettable capillaries were filled by a
syringe. The capillary was allowed to equilibrate with
the prostaglandin solution for two minutes before sealing. The ends of the capillary tubes were sealed by in-
serting a nylon rod dipped in Eastman 910 adhesive. After waiting for a few minutes for the adhesive to dry,
the ends were carefully coated with an overseal of 10%
cellulose acetate solution in methyl-ethyl-ketone. Immediately after sealing, the capillary fiber was inserted
into a U-tube and then placed in a humid atmosphere for
one day prior to testing in order to assure permeation
of the prostaglandin into the capsule walls. After overnight equilibration, the U-tube was filled with 1.4 ml
of dialysate solution (pH 7.4 phosphate buffer) and
then placed in a Dubnoff shaker at 37°. Stirring was
accomplished at a frequency of 36 cycles per minute. At
the end of the prescribed collection period, the dialysate was quantitatively transferred to a counting vial,
containing the scintillation fluid. Fresh dialysate

Table II.   Release of $PGF_{2\alpha}$ from Capillary Microcapsules

Capillary Material*	Capillary Dimensions, mils		Fractional Release, Q_t/Q_o, at Time, t, hr					
	O.D.	I.D.	0.1	0.5	1	3	6	24
Cellulose acetate (phthalate plasticizer)	18	15	0	0	0	0	0	0
Cellulose acetate (citrate plasticizer)	14	12	0.01	0.02	0.04	0.07	0.13	0.17
Deacetylated cellulose acetate	12	9	0.60	0.94	0.99	0.99	0.99	1.0
Cellulose butyrate	17	15	0.01	0.01	0.01	0.01	0.02	0.02
Ethyl cellulose	18	15	0.01	0.02	0.03	0.04	0.05	0.05
Nylon 6,6	13	10	0.01	0.03	0.06	0.12	0.20	0.41
Silicone polycarbonate	17	14	0.05	0.06	0.07	0.08	0.09	0.10
Silicone rubber	37	20	0.02	0.03	0.03	0.04	0.04	0.05

*Cellulose acetate, Eastman, 33% diethyl phthalate; cellulose acetate, Eastman, 34% acetyl triethyl citrate; cellulose butyrate, Eastman, diethyl phthalate; ethyl cellulose, American Polymers; nylon 6,6, Du Pont, Zytel 101; silicone polycarbonate, General Electric, MEM; silicone, Dow Corning, Silastic 602-135.

was then added and samples were collected at 5 minutes,
30 minutes, 1, 3, 6, and 24 hours. After removal of the
24-hour dialysate sample, the capsule was broken and its
contents analyzed for residual radioactive prostaglandin. The counts obtained in the dialysate were divided
by the total counts of all the dialysates and the capsule.

    Capillary dimensions are means of ten readings. The
capillaries were encapsulated in silicone rubber, and
measurements were made on cross sections under the
microscope.

    The water tolerance test was adopted for estimat-
ing the acetyl content of the cellulose acetate capsule
material. This method was described by Malm et al.[19]
A known weight of capsule material was dissolved in 10
ml of acetone and titrated with water until a precipi-
tate formed. To improve the determination of the end
point, the absorption of the solution was measured at
380 mm using a Bausch and Lomb Spectronic 20. An
absorbance reading of 0.1 was used for the water toler-
ance value.

IV.   IN VITRO TEST RESULTS

Preliminary Studies

    In the initial tests, $PGF_{2\alpha}$ diffusion rates were
determined on several types of polymers in the form of
capillaries. Seven different materials were examined.
The dimensions of the capillaries and the results of the
permeability measurements are presented in Table II. In
general, the more swellable or hydrated polymers seem to
give the higher prostaglandin permeability. This would
be anticipated since prostaglandin is ionized at physiological pH.

    Although many polymers could be tested to achieve
a diffusion of prostaglandin intermediate between deacetylated cellulose acetate and other polymers, we
elected to modify cellulose acetate. Secondary control
of release rates could be achieved by changing the fiber
geometry.

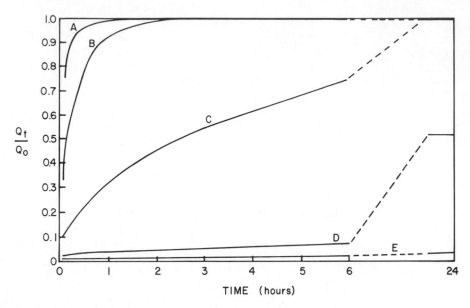

Figure 2.   Permeability of $PGF_{2\alpha}$ across modified cellu-
             lose acetate membranes. A, deacetylated;
             B and C, partially deacetylated by treatment
             with 0.34 and 0.17 g/l, respectively, of
             sodium hydroxide in methanol for one hour at
             room temperature; D, deplasticized by treat-
             ment with methanol only; and E, untreated.

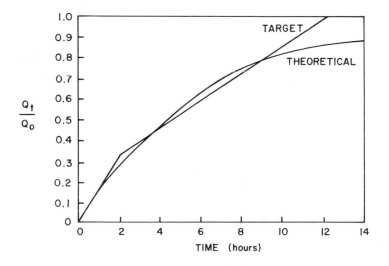

Figure 3.   Comparison between target dose rate curve and
             theoretical diffusion curve.

Modification of Cellulose Acetate

Cellulose acetate was too impermeable to be of any practical value in this study, and completely deacetylated cellulose acetate was too permeable. A study was therefore made of the permeability of the partially deacetylated and deplasticized polymer. Cellulose acetate capillaries were partially de-esterified by treatment with 0.17 g/liter and 0.34 g/liter methanolic sodium hydroxide for one hour at room temperature. The data are shown in Figure 2. The permeability of a completely deacetylated capillary is also shown. It is evident that different prostaglandin permeabilities can be obtained by changing the acetyl content of the cellulose molecule. The effect of deacetylation on cellulose acetate permeability is well known. The results of the 0.17 g/liter sodium hydroxide treated capillaries were replotted in order to permit calculation of the diffusion coefficient. The values obtained for D are 0.8 and 1.9 x 10^{-7} cm/sec. The equation is:

$$D = \frac{r_i^2 \ln \frac{r_o}{r_i}}{2} \; \frac{2.3 \, \Delta\log(1 - Q_t/Q_o)}{\Delta t}$$

Correlation with Target Dose Rate

Figure 3 is a comparison between the target delivery dose rate as recommended by Professor Sultan Karim, and the theoretical curve calculated from diffusion constants obtained with a capillary microcapsule containing a solution of $PGF_{2\alpha}$ THAM salt. Except for the last two hours, there is good approximation between the two profiles. This desired rate of permeation of prostaglandin (data points at 1, 3, and 6 hours) was achieved by treatment of cellulose acetate capillaries with methanolic sodium hydroxide at pH 11.9.

Effect of System Variables

The influence of several system variables on the relative diffusion of prostaglandins through modified cellulose acetate membranes was studied. The effect of deplasticization was pronounced.

In the initial studies with small diameter capillaries, diffusion of prostaglandin was only about 1% in 6 hours for the untreated fiber. With deacetylation in

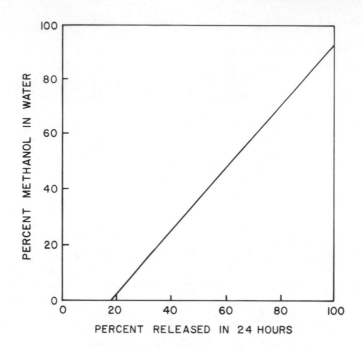

Figure 4.   Effect of methanol concentration in the cellu-
             lose acetate deplasticization bath on the re-
             lease of prostaglandin from the capsules.

100% methanol only 7% diffused in 6 hours (Figure 4).
Studies with larger diameter capsules, containing a different plasticizer, indicated that this plasticized
fiber was quite permeable.   Partial removal of the
citrate plasticizer was then attempted with aqueous
methanol (Figure 4).   From this study it was concluded
that removal of plasticizer is very effective in changing the diffusion properties of the capsules.   No attempt
was made to compare the effect of different plasticizers
on the permeability of the polymer.

     However, several other changes had little or no ef-
fect.   They include changes in stirring rate, dialysate
concentration, type of prostaglandin salt (PGE_1 or
$PGF_{2\alpha}$) and the concentration and pH of prostaglandin
solution.   These studies will be briefly discussed.

Since the prostaglandin salt is extremely soluble in water, there is a large concentration gradient across the membrane. A small concentration in a stagnant layer outside the capsule was not expected to be a problem. The rate of shaker oscillation was changed from 36 to 60 rpm without changing the diffusion, as shown in Table III.

The effect of dialysate ionic strength was investigated. The normal dialysate composition was chosen to simulate vaginal fluid pH and ionic strength.[20] In our studies we have compared the diffusion of $PGF_{2\alpha}$ in the buffer mentioned above; ten times this concentration; and pure water. The data, shown in Table IV, do not indicate any effect of dialysate concentration on diffusion.

The diffusion coefficient, including the solubility factor, was relatively unaffected by the prostaglandin concentration. Also the diffusion of $PGF_{2\alpha}$ and PGE_1 was found to be similar. This would be anticipated since the molecular size and solubility are similar. Supporting data are shown in Table V.

The possible precipitation of prostaglandins by the acid conditions in the vagina, and the complexing of prostaglandin by components of the vaginal and uterine fluids, have been considered. Under acid conditions, prostaglandins are quite insoluble. This factor could affect diffusion since the prostaglandin crystal must dissolve before the prostaglandin can diffuse through the capillary wall.

The PGE_1 (THAM) was prepared, as described before, by adding THAM to a suspension of PGE_1. The pH of this solution was varied from pH 6 to 9. There was no apparent effect of pH after one day storage (standard procedure) as shown in Table VI.

V. IN VIVO EVALUATION

Sixteen microcapsules of various sizes were implanted in the rabbit vagina. Eleven others were implanted subcutaneously in the rabbit back. These tests were performed with two capillaries with 0.35/0.30 OD/ID and 1.4/1.2 OD/ID. Some capsules contained PGE_1 and others $PGF_{2\alpha}$. The early tests used 1 mg of prostaglandin. However, since the biological response was minimal, later tests were performed with larger quantities of prosta-

Table III. Effect of Dialysate
Flow on Diffusion

Oscillation rpm	Diffusion in 6 hours, %	
36	60 ± 1	N = 2
60	62 ± 1	N = 2

Table IV. Effect of Dialysate
Concentration on Diffusion

Dialysate	Diffusion in 3 hours, %	
H_2O	72 ± 6	N = 4
Buffer	66 ± 12	N = 6
10X Buffer	72 ± 14	N = 2

Table V. Effect of PG Type and
Concentration on Diffusion

Fiber Type	PG	Conc.	No.	Diffusion in 3 hours, %
Type 1	E_1	<0.5%	2	54 ± 10
	E_1	1/1	8	59 ± 11
Type 2	E_1	0.5%	2	44 ± 22
	$F_{2\alpha}$	0.5%	2	38 ± 6

Table VI. Effect of Prostaglandin pH on Diffusion

pH	Diffusion in 3 hours, %	
6	76 ± 0	N = 2
8	69 ± 4	N = 2
9	78 ± 12	N = 3

Table VII.   Rabbit Response to Intravaginal Implants

	PGE_1					$PGF_{2\alpha}$			
Capsule content (mg)	3	4	8	10	20	3	4	8	20
No. of Implants	1	1	2	3	4	1	1	1	2
No. of Responses				2	3	1	1		2
Average Response (minutes)				95	156	60	80		103

Table VIII.   Rabbit Response to Subcutaneous Implants

	PGE_1			$PGF_{2\alpha}$			
Capsule content (mg)	3	4	8	1	2	3	8
No. Implanted	1	1	3	1	1	2	2
No of Responses	1		1		1	1	1
Average Response (minutes)	60		90		60	60	240

glandin (4, 8, 10, and 20 mg PG THAM salt).   The biological activity of the capsules was monitored by measuring changes in the oviduct or uterine contractile pressure.   The PGE_1 inhibits oviduct motility and the $PGF_{2\alpha}$
stimulates it.   The results are presented in Tables VII
and VIII.

The effect of increased prostaglandin levels is
demonstrated in both types of PG as an increase in the
number of implants showing activity and as an increase
in the response period.   The need for such high levels
of prostaglandin was unexpected since the total target
dose in the human was only 15 mg/14 hours.   However,
recent reports by Karim seem to indicate that in humans

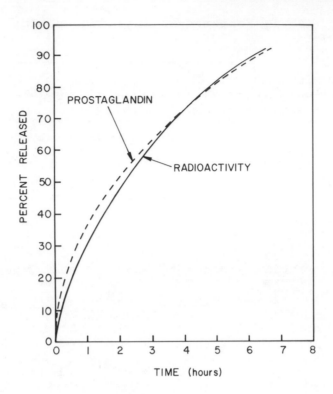

Figure 5.   In vitro release of PGF$_{2\alpha}$ from capillary
            microcapsules analyzed by direct counting
            and radioimmunoassay.

an abortion was obtained by the intravaginal route after
nearly 300 mg of PGF$_{2\alpha}$ was given divided into six intervals of 2-1/2 hours each.[21] It is also reported that
prostaglandins seem to lose 20-30% of their activity
when implanted in the vagina.

     To prove that the prostaglandin was not changed dur-
ing the encapsulation procedure, a radioimmunoassay procedure was used to measure the prostaglandin in the
dialysate. The results (Figure 5) established that the
analysis of radioactivity in the dialysate did measure
prostaglandin diffusion and not that of a radioactive
metabolite.

     Twelve capsules were retrieved from the rabbit and
their contents analyzed for residual prostaglandin. Approximately 20% of their content remained in the capsule.

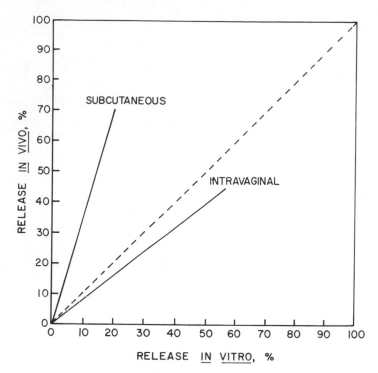

Figure 6.   Comparison between _in vitro_ and _in vivo_ re-
             lease rates in two different locations in
             the body.   Least-square slopes are drawn
             for each location.   Dashed line is 45°
             theoretical line for perfect correlation.

The data are presented in Figure 6.   The best lines (vis-
ual) were drawn for the subcutaneous and intravaginal
implants.   In addition, the 1:1 correlation line is
shown.   The release rates of the subcutaneous implants
seem to be slower than the _in vitro_ results indicate.
This is attributed to the presence of additional mass
transport resistance in the tissue.   Similar resistance
was reported by Kincl and Rudel.[22]   On the other hand,
the release rate of the intravaginal implants seems to
have been slightly accelerated.   It is not possible to
speculate about the causes of this.   Conflicting results
have been reported in the literature.   Sundaram and
Kincl[4] observed a similar enhancement in release rate of
steroids when he changed his dialysate from saline to

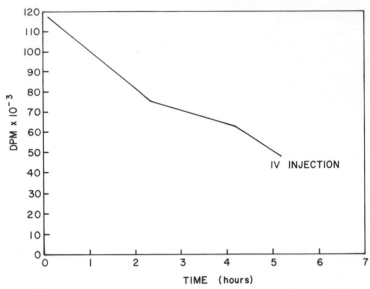

Figure 7.   Plasma radioactivity level after intravenous
             $PGF_{2\alpha}$ injection.

plasma. He attributed this to the effect plasma lipids
had on the silicone membrane. Yet Croxatto et al.[11]
reported that contraceptive effectiveness of the implants
lasted about one-third the time predicted from in vitro
measurements. Further studies will be required to con-
firm these observations. We also examined the fate of
prostaglandin $PGF_{2\alpha}$ after intravenous injection. The
results shown in Figure 7 indicate that the blood levels
of $PGF_{2\alpha}$ and/or its metabolites are reduced by 60% in
five hours. Comparison of this result with capsule implant and infusion experiments should allow calculation
of the in vivo capsule permeation.

VI.   ACKNOWLEDGMENTS

     This program was supported by a subcontract with
the Worcester Foundation for Experimental Biology under
the terms of their Contract No. AID/csd 2837 with the
Agency for International Development. We wish to thank
Dr. Michael J. K. Harper formerly at the Worcester
Foundation and currently Medical Officer at the World
Health Organization; and Dr. Richard P. de Filippi,
Vice President of Research and Development at Abcor,
Inc. for valuable discussions during the course of this
work. We also would like to thank Dr. C. Spillman for
the in vivo studies.

REFERENCES

1. L. L. Doyle and T. H. Clewe, _Amer. J. Obstet. Gynec._, __101__, 564 (1968).

2. D. R. Mishell and M. E. Lumkin, _Fertil. and Steril._, __21__, 99 (1970).

3. F. A. Kincl, G. Benagiano, and I. Angee, _Steroids_, __11__, 673 (1968).

4. D. Sundaram and F. A. Kincl, _Steroids_, __12__, 517 (1968).

5. C. C. Chang and F. A. Kincl, _Steroids_, __12__, 689 (1968).

6. C. C. Chang and F. A. Kincl, _Fertil. and Steril._, __21__, 134 (1970).

7. A. S. Lifchez and A. Scommegna, _Fertil. and Steril._, __21__, 426 (1970).

8. A. Scommegna, G. N. Pandya, M. Christ, A. W. Lee, and M. R. Cohen, _Fertil. and Steril._, __21__, 201 (1970).

9. M. R. Cohen, G. N. Pandya, and A. Scommegna, _Fertil. and Steril._, __21__, 715 (1970).

10. P. J. Dziuk and B. Cook, _Endocrinology_, __78__, 208 (1966).

11. H. B. Croxatto, S. Diaz, P. Atria, S. Cheviakoff, S. Rosatti, and H. Oddo, _Contraception_, __4__, 155 (1971).

12. C. F. Most, _J. Biomed. Mater. Res._, __6__, 3 (1972).

13. J. C. Fu, A. K. Kale, and D. L. Moyer, _J. Biomed. Mater. Res._, __7__, 71 (1973).

14. R. L. Shippy, S. Hwang, and R. G. Bung, _J. Biomed. Mater. Res._, __7__, 95 (1973).

15. N. Wiqvist, M. Bygdeman, and M. Toppozada, _Research in Prostaglandins_, __2__, No. 3, Worcester Foundation for Experimental Biology, 1972.

16. S. Bergstrom and B. Samuelsson, Ann. Rev. Biochem.,
     34, 101 (1965).

17. S. H. Ferreira and J. R. Vane, Nature, 216, 868
     (1967).

18. J. Crank, "The Mathematics of Diffusion", Oxford
     University Press, London, 1956, p. 62.

19. C. J. Malm, L. J. Tanghe, B. C. Laird, and G. D.
     Smith, J. Am. Chem. Soc., 75, 80 (1953).

20. D. Olds and N. L. Van Demark, Fertil. and Steril.,
     8, 345 (1957).

21. S. M. M. Karim and S. D. Sharma, J. Obstet. Gynec.
     (Brit. Comwlth.), 78, 294 (1971).

22. F. A. Kincl and H. W. Rudel, Acta Endocrinol.
     (Copenhagen) Suppl., 151 (1971).

CERVICAL HYDROGEL DILATOR: A NEW DELIVERY

SYSTEM FOR PROSTAGLANDINS

M. K. Akkapeddi and B. D. Halpern
Polysciences, Inc.
Warrington, Pennsylvania 18976
        and
R. H. Davis and H. Balin
Hahneman Medical College and Hospital
Philadelphia, Pennsylvania 19102

I. INTRODUCTION

The prostaglandins are becoming increasingly important with a variety of possible therapeutic applications. One focus of current interest is their role in reproductive physiology for potential application in fertility control. Prostaglandins PGE_2 and $PGF_{2\alpha}$ have been shown to be effective for induction of therapeutic abortions in humans when administered by various routes[1-4] such as intravenous, intrauterine, and intravaginal routes. The rapid metabolic degradation of prostaglandins necessitates a dosage schedule of repeated administrations or continuous infusion until abortion is induced. However, this results in the systemic circulation of prostaglandins and their metabolites and causes concomitant side effects such as diarrhea, nausea, and pyrexia. Since the primary role of PGE_2 and $PGF_{2\alpha}$ in the induction of abortion is the stimulation of uterine smooth muscle causing the necessary uterine contractions, it would be more desirable to apply the drugs at the target organ, viz., the uterus. It has indeed been shown that direct intrauterine instillation[2,3] of prostaglandins <u>via</u> a catheter is effective at lower doses, although the method needed further simplification. In this regard, sustained release of the drug from a polymer matrix becomes a convenient approach. In our cervical hydrogel dilator

delivery method, the prostaglandin is released from the
matrix of a swellable, hydrophilic polymer inserted at
the cervix uteri, where it serves the dual purpose of
cervical dilation and controlled release of the drug at
the uterus. The cervical dilation is caused by the
swelling of the polymer in the uterine/cervical fluids
and its action is similar to that of "laminaria tents"
used in current clinical practice.[5] The slow and gradual cervical dilation so obtained seems to have some
advantages over the use of mechanical aids such as Hegar,
Goodell, and vibratory-type dilators commonly used in
the surgical D&C procedure. For example, the rapid
mechanical dilation of cervix may in some cases result
in a clinical syndrome called cervical incompetence.[6]
Our initial studies were directed towards the use of
synthetic, swellable hydrophilic polymers as cervical
dilators. However, for a therapeutic abortion, uterine
evacuation is necessary in addition to cervical dilation
and hence we have studied the use of prostaglandins via
this delivery method.

II. MATERIALS AND METHODS

Monomers and Polymers

α,ω-Polyethylene glycol diacrylates (PEGDA) and
dimethacrylates (PEGDMA) of different molecular weights
were made by the transesterification of polyethylene
glycols of narrow molecular-weight distribution, and
ethyl acrylate or methyl methacrylate, with tetra-
isopropyl titanate (TPT) as catalyst.

$$HO(CH_2CH_2O)_nH + CH_2=CCOO\,R' \xrightarrow[TPT]{-R'OH} CH_2=CCOO(CH_2CH_2O)_nCOC=CH_2$$

$$I$$

$$R = H,\ CH_3$$
$$n = 80,\ 150,\ 500$$

These long-chain compounds were either homopolymerized
(self crosslinked) or copolymerized with other monomers
such as acrylamide or acrylamidoglucose.

2-Acrylamidoglucose was prepared by selective
N-acrylation of glucosamine.

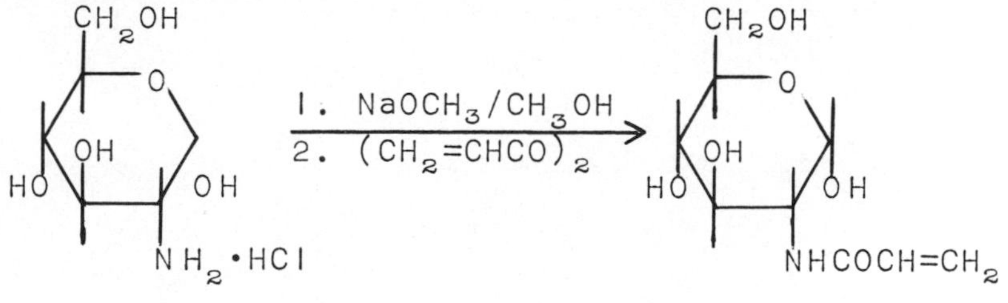

II

6-O-Methacrylylgalactose was prepared from D-galactose
by the procedure of Black et al.[7]

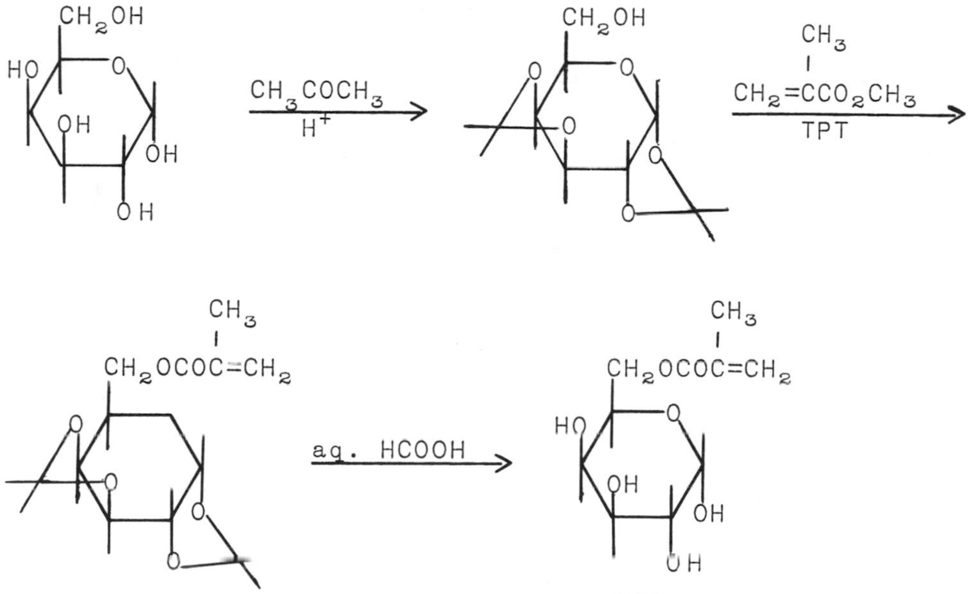

III

These monomers (II and III) were polymerized with methylene bis-acrylamide (MBA) or PEGDA 4000 as crosslinking
agents. All of the hydrogels were made in aqueous system
with the redox catalyst, ammonium persulfate/tetramethyl-
ethylenediamine. After purification by repeated dialysis
in water, they were dried in air and vacuum. They were
then allowed to absorb a known amount of prostaglandin
solutions and finally dried in a stream of dry nitrogen
followed by vacuum to predetermined cylindrically shaped
rods. The prostaglandins PGE_2 and $PGF_{2\alpha}$ required for
this purpose were converted to the respective trometh-
amine salts and used.

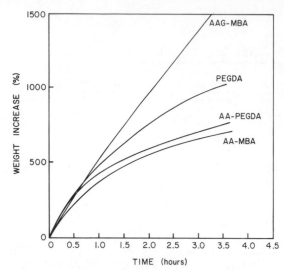

Figure 1.   Rates of swelling of hydrogels in water.   Com-
             positions, initial solids content of gels, and
             weight increases at equilibrium are the follow-
             ing: 2-acrylamidoglucose-methylenebisacryl-
             amide (AAG-MBA), 6%, 4100%; acrylamide-
             methylenebisacrylamide (AA-MBA), 5%, 2400%;
             polyethylene glycol 4000 diacrylate (PEGDA),
             10%, 1200%; and acrylamide-polyethylene
             glycol 4000 diacrylate (1:1 n/w) (AA-PEGDA),
             3%, 2500%.

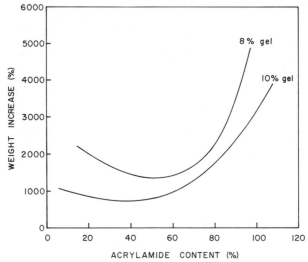

Figure 2.   Effects of acrylamide content on weight in-
             creases in water at equilibrium (14 days) of
             AA-PEGDA 6000 gels.   The gel values (8% and
             10%) are the solids contents before dehydra-
             tion and immersion.

Cervical Dilation

Adult pregnant (12 days) New Zealand White rabbits were anesthetized by I.P. Nembutal (15-30 mg/kg body wt.) plus ether by cone. The abdomen was opened and a small transvaginal incision was made. The hydrophilic polymer rod (4 mm in diameter) containing prostaglandin was inserted into one of the cervices of the two uterine horns. Each animal was observed over a period of 24-72 hours for abortion effect.

III. RESULTS AND DISCUSSION

Polymer Properties

Several generalizations were drawn from studies of the swelling behavior of these polymers. First, homopolymers of polyethylene glycol diacrylate (PEGDA) or dimethacrylate (PEGDMA) showed an increase in water absorption with an increase in chain length from PEG 4000 to PEG 20,000. Second, polymers derived from acrylamidoglucose or methacrylylgalactose showed not only high swellability but also high rates of hydration (Figure 1); however, these gels were in general weak. And third, copolymers derived from PEGDA or PEGDMA with other monomers, such as acrylamide (AA) or acrylamidoglucose (AAG), in general had good strength. They showed increased swellability with increase in the ratio of AA (or AAG) to PEGDA but showed a minimum at an approximate weight ratio of the comonomers of 1:1 (Figure 2). Conversely, the strength of the gels appeared to be the highest at a comonomer ratio of about 1:1. This is probably due to an interchain attraction between polyacrylamide or polyacrylamidoglucose and polyether segments of the molecules involving hydrogen bonding. So choice of the polymers had to be optimized between mechanical strength and swellability which are mutually conflicting properties.

Cervical Dilation in Rabbits

Our extensive studies in rabbits showed that considerable cervical dilation can be obtained with the polymers alone, although with no abortion effect. Some of the data are shown in Table I. Histopathologic studies of cervical tissue exposed to these polymers

Table I. Polymer-Induced Cervical Dilation of Adult New Zealand White Rabbits

Polymer Composition Monomer(s)*	Solids, %***	In Vitro Swelling, %****	In Vivo Increase in Cervical Diameter, %
AA (0.08% MBA, 0.5% agarose)	5	1840	165 (24 hr – non-pregnant)
AA (0.08% MBA)	8	1540 (24 hr)	115 (3 hr – non-pregnant)
PEGDA 4000	10	1200	228 (24 hr – 12-day pregnant)
AA-PEGDA 4000 (6:1 w/w)	5	2500	175 (24 hr – 12-day pregnant)
AA-PEGDA 4000 (1:1 w/w)	2	3000	300 (72 hr – 12-day pregnant)
AAG (0.05% MBA)	5	3900	292 (72 hr – 12-day pregnant)
AAG-PEGDA 4000 (2:1 w/w)	5	1900	360 (72 hr – 12-day pregnant)
AA-PEGDA 6000 (1:1 w/w)	3	2325	273.5 (24 hr – 28-day pregnant)
AA-PEGDA 6000 (1:1 w/w)	4	1650	177 (24 hr – 28-day pregnant)

*Acrylamide (AA); methylenebisacrylamide (MBA); polyethylene glycol 4000/6000 diacrylate (PEGDA 4000/6000); and 2-acrylamidoglucose (AAG). **Before dehydration. ***Weight increase at equilibrium.

showed no tissue damage or local reaction indicating that
these materials are biocompatible.

Controlled Delivery of Prostaglandins

Since prostaglandins need a controlled target organ
application to minimize side effects, a cervical hydrogel
dilator delivery system seemed to be a suitable choice.
Accordingly we studied the effectiveness of prostaglandins
incorporated in the hydrogels for the induction of abortion in 12-day pregnant New Zealand White rabbits. The
results of the in vivo experiments are summarized in
Tables II and III. Excellent abortion was noted with as
low as 2 mg of $PGF_{2\alpha}$-tromethamine salt (equivalent to
about 1.5 mg $PGF_{2\alpha}$) incorporated in the polymer, especially when the latter had good swellability. This is in
marked contrast to the minimum dosage of 21 mg $PGF_{2\alpha}$
which is closer to the toxic levels reported by Chang et
al.,[8] for the induction of abortion in rabbits by subcutaneous injections. Also these workers reported that
no abortion effect was found with even 20 mg $PGF_{2\alpha}$ in a
Silastic capsule implanted under the skin of the pregnant
rabbit, indicating that either the release of the drug
was insufficient or not reaching the uterus in the required levels. Our results indicate that the prostaglandins are released at the uterus in sufficient levels,
while at the same time the cervical dilation due to polymer swelling has an apparent synergistic effect, inasmuch
as the effective dose levels are reduced to nearly 1/20
that of other routes of administration. The results with
PGE_2 were similar, although seemingly less effective than
reported in literature, and indicate the need to choose
a more stable salt of PGE_2.

It may be pointed out that a hydrogel is particularly
suited to "short term" sustained release of drugs such as
is the case with prostaglandins. It needs low load of
the drug in the polymer because of high rate of diffusion,
especially if the drug is adequately soluble in the body
fluids. This is in contrast to Silastic, which although
suitable for long term sustained delivery, is probably
not effective for short term application, unless a large
reservoir of the drug is encapsulated or a large amount
of the drug is incorporated in the polymer, as is evident
from Chang's work.

Theoretical derivations and subsequent experimental
work of T. Higuchi,[9] Roseman,[10] etc., showed that the
fraction (F) of the total amount of drug released from

Table II. The Abortifacient Effect of Prostaglandin $F_{2\alpha}$ on 12-Day Pregnant New Zealand White Rabbits when Administered by Cervical Polymer Plug

Polymer Composition Monomer(s)*	Solids, %***	In Vitro swelling, %****	Dose in the Polymer, mg*****	Abortions Hr	A/N******	Abortive Effect
AA (0.08% MBA, 0.5% agarose)	5	1700	1.0	24	0/13	no
AAG (0.18% MBA)	8	2200	2.0	72	11/11	yes
AAG (0.07% MBA)	6	5300	2.0	72	11/11	yes
AAG-PEGDA 4000 (1:1 w/w)	4	1200	3.0	72	0/11	no
AA-PEGDA 4000 (6:1 w/w)	4	1800	3.0	72	9/9	yes
AAG-PEGDA 4000 (1:1 w/w)	6	1500	3.5	48	12/12	yes
AAG (0.05% MBA)	5	4400	4.0	72	11/11	yes
AA-PEGDA 4000 (5:1 w/w)	2	3000	5.6	26	14/14	yes
AAG-PEGDA 4000 (1:1 w/w)	6	1500	6.0	48	12/12	yes

*Acrylamide (AA); methylenebisacrylamide (MBA); 2-acrylamidoglucose (AAG); and polyethylene glycol 4000 diacrylate (PEGDA 4000). **Before dehydration. ***Weight increase when immersed 3-5 days in water. ****PGF$_{2\alpha}$-salt was Prostaglandin $F_{2\alpha}$-Tromethamine salt (all except first case). *****A/N = no. aborted/total no. of fetuses.

Table III. The Abortifacient Effect of Prostaglandin E2 on 12-Day Pregnant New Zealand White Rabbits when Administered by Cervical Polymer Plug

| Polymer Composition | | In Vitro Swelling, %**** | Dose in the Polymer, mg***** | Abortions | | Abortive Effect |
Monomer(s)*	Solids, %***			Hr	A/N******	
AAG-PEGDA 4000 (1:1 w/w)	5	1200	1.2	72	0/8	no
AAG-PEGDA 4000 (1:2 w/w)	8	1300	2.0	120	2/12	yes
AA-PEGDA 4000 (5:1 w/w)	2.5	2900	2.0	72	2/8	yes
AAG-PEGDA 4000 (2:1 w/w)	4	1900	2.4	72	0/14	no
AAG (0.2% MBA)	5	3900	2.7	72	4/4	yes
AAG-PEGDA 4000 (1:2 w/w)	6	1050	4.0	48	0/7	no
AAG (0.2% MBA)	5	3900	4.2	72	7/9	yes
AAG-PEGDA 4000 (2:1 w/w)	5	1900	4.5	72	10/10	yes
AA-PEGDA 4000 (5:1 w/w)	2.5	2900	5.2	72	2/5	yes
AA-PEGDA 4000 (5:1 w/w)	3.0	3000	5.8	72	8/10	yes
AAG (0.2% MBA)	5	3900	8.1	72	6/11	yes

*Acrylamide (AA); methylenebisacrylamide (MBA); 2-acrylamidoglucose (AAG); and polyethylene glycol 4000 diacrylate (PEGDA 4000). **Before dehydration. ***Weight increase when immersed 3-5 days in water. ****PGE$_2$-salt was Prostaglandin E$_2$-Tromethamine salt (all except first case). *****A/N = no. aborted/total no. of fetuses.

a cylindrical matrix follows the kinetic equation:

$$\left[\frac{F}{4} + \frac{1-F}{4} \ln(1-F) \right]^{\frac{1}{2}} = kt^{\frac{1}{2}}$$

where

$$k = \left(\frac{C_m D_m}{W} \right)^{\frac{1}{2}} r$$

and C_m is the solubility of the drug in the matrix (mg cm^{-3}), D_m is the diffusion coefficient for the drug in the matrix, W is the concentration of drug in the matrix (mg cm^{-3}), r is the radius of the cylinder (cm), and t is time (sec).

For a nonswelling polymer, a plot of F vs t is approximately a parabolic curve, i.e., $F \propto t^{\frac{1}{2}}$. For a swelling polymer, the relationship is more complex, particularly when the rate of swelling is not rapid, as normally expected in vivo due to the limited availability of cervical fluids. As the polymer swells, the value of "k" increases, since r, D_m, and C_m/W increase with time. If $K \propto t^x$, we would then get an approximate relationship $F \propto t^{\left(\frac{1}{2}+x\right)}$ where x>0. This means that the rate of release of drug does not decline with time, as in the case of nonswelling polymer, but may either be constant ($x=\frac{1}{2}$) or increase with time ($x>\frac{1}{2}$) until either the drug is completely exhausted or the polymer has attained equilibrium swelling whichever is earlier (Figure 3). In the case of a highly swellable polymer ($x>>\frac{1}{2}$) the drug is released very rapidly after the polymer attains a certain degree of hydration. By modifying the polymer structure and method of formation, the degree and rate of swellability may be optimized to desirable results, viz., constancy of release rate. However, the applicability of this system would be limited by the "equilibrium swelling time" of the polymer and hence useful for only short term release of drugs such as prostaglandins.

Thus, in summary, the cervical route of administration of prostaglandin in a "hydrogel dilator vehicle has the following advantages:

(1) Low dosage rates (1/20 of that by other routes in rabbits)

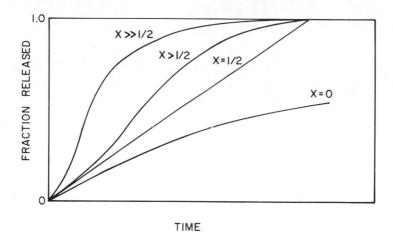

Figure 3.   Predicted behavior of rates of release of a
             drug from a cylindrical matrix (nonswelling
             <u>vs</u> swelling polymers).

(2)   Apparent synergestic action of cervical
dilation by polymer swelling and uterine con-
traction (by prostaglandins)

(3)   Proximity to target organs, with less chance
of metabolic degradation and systemic side effects.

(4)   Relatively simple procedure of administration.

(5)   Easy manipulation of polymer properties according to the requirements (polymerization parameters
allow multiple variations).

(6)   Possibility of obtaining constant drug release
rate with minimum drug load in the polymer.

(7)   Gradual dilation less likely to result in
possible cervical trauma and subsequent internal
os cervical incompetence.

ACKNOWLEDGMENT

This work was supported by N.I.H. Contract 71/2239.

REFERENCES

1. C. H. Hendricks, W. E. Brenner, L. Ekbladh,
    V. Brotanek, and J. I. Fishburne, Jr., Amer. J.
    Obstet. Gynec., 111, 564 (1971).

2. M. P. Embrey and E. Hillier, Brit. Med. J., 1,
    588 (1971).

3. M. T. Toppozada, M. Bygdeman, and N. Wyquist,
    Contraception, 4, 293 (1971).

4. S. M. M. Karim and S. D. Sharma, J. Obstet. Gynec.
    Brit. Comm., 78 294 (1971).

5. R. W. Hale and R. J. Pion, Clinical Obstetrics and
    Gynecology, 15, No. 3, (Sept. 1972).

6. C. S. W. Wright et al., Lancet, 3, 1278 (1972).

7. W. A. P. Black, J. A. Colquhoun, and E. T. Dewar,
    Makromol. Chem., 117, 210 (1968).

8. M. C. Chang and D. M. Hunt, Nature, 236, 120 (1972).

9. T. Higuchi, J. Pharm. Sci., 52, 1145 (1963).

10. T. J. Roseman, J. Pharm. Sci., 61, 46 (1972).

LONG-ACTING DELIVERY SYSTEMS FOR NARCOTIC ANTAGONISTS

S. Yolles, John Eldridge, Thomas Leafe, and
J. H. R. Woodland
University of Delaware
Newark, Delaware 197111
        and
David R. Blake* and Francis Meyer**
University of Maryland
Baltimore, Maryland 21201

I. INTRODUCTION

The development of systems for delivering narcotic
antagonists and other drugs, such as steroids, to
patients at a controlled rate over a long period of time,
perhaps months, has been the object of investigations by
this laboratory for the last four years. The system at
present under study comprises incorporating the drug in
a plastic matrix, shaping the composite into a convenient
form, such as films, pellets or chips, and then implanting the structure into the body tissue of animals by
surgery or hypodermic injection. The drug migrates continuously from the interior of the polymeric composite
to the outer surface, where it is dissolved or swept
away by the body fluid surrounding the structure. The
mechanism of this migration through the polymer is that
of diffusion and the driving force is the concentration
gradient.[1-3]

Although the concept of delivering from a depot has
been described,[4] the earlier systems comprised a compact
mixture of polymer and drug in granular form, having open

---

*Present address: School of Medicine, Johns Hopkins,
  Baltimore, Md. 21205.
**Present address: Extracorporeal Medical Specialties,
  Inc., King of Prussia, Pa. 19406

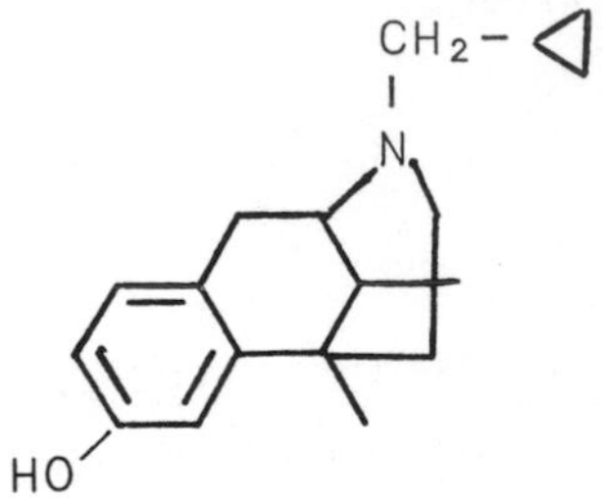

Figure 1.   Chemical Structures of Narcotic Antagonists

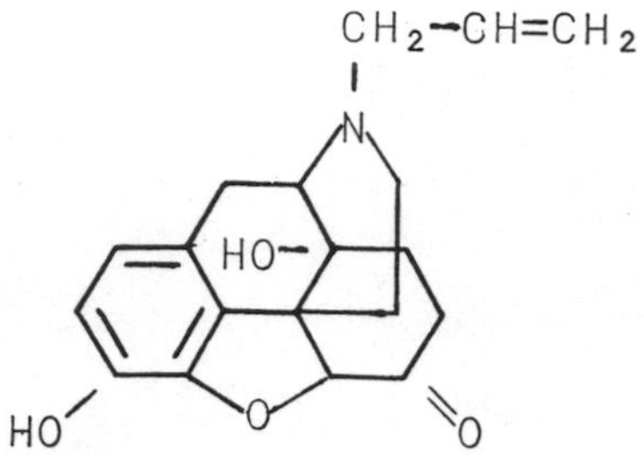

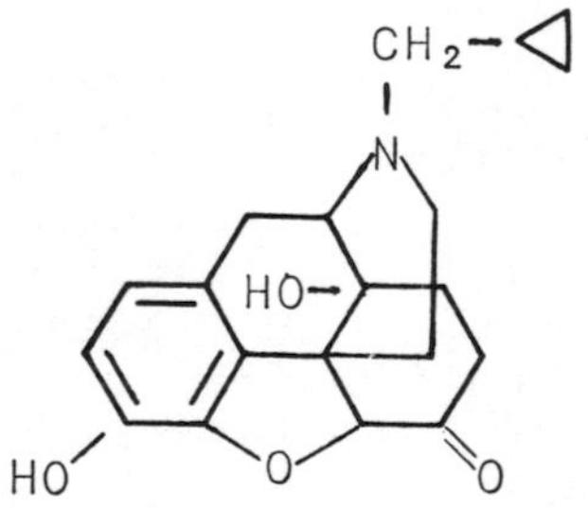

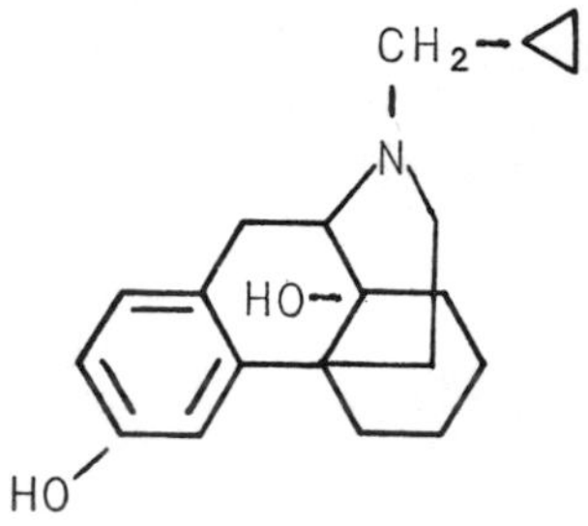

channels between the grains. In this case, the drug was
leached by fluid which penetrated these channels. In our
drug-polymer composites, the drug must migrate by diffusion through the polymer walls.

II. MATERIALS AND METHODS

In the present work, the composites were prepared by
melt-pressing into sheets a mixture of morphine antagonist (some of which was tritiated), polymer, and plasticizer at 145° under one metric ton load for 10 seconds
and using shims of thickness varying from 0.40 to 0.91
mm. Most of the studies were carried out with three
narcotic antagonists: cyclazocine (2-cyclopropylmethyl-
2'-hydroxy-5,9-dimethyl-6,7-benzomorphan); naltrexone
(17-cyclopropylmethyl-4,5α-epoxy-3,14-dihydroxymorphinan-
6-one); and naloxone (17-allyl-4,5α-epoxy-3,14-dihydroxy-
morphinan-6-one). A structurally related antagonist,
ℓ-BC-2605 (ℓ-1-N-cyclopropylmethyl-3,14-dihydroxy-
morphinan), is now being investigated. The chemical
structures of all four are shown in Figure 1. Generally,
the composites contained 20% of the drug, but recently
some contained more, e.g., 35%. The film thus obtained
was either used as such, in samples of 4 cm^2, or was reduced to small particles and screened, fractions falling
within sieves Nos. 25/35, 40/60, or 35/70 (0.71/0.5,
0.42/0.25, or 0.5/0.21 mm). The specific radioactivities
of the samples were determined by combustion of the polymer matrices and radioassaying the water trapped in a
Tricarb Oxidizer System. The efficacy of these composites was determined by measuring the release rates of
the antagonist in vivo (rats) and in vitro and by the
physiological response in dogs and in mice.

In experiments in vivo, the delivery rates of the
antagonist were determined by surgically implanting or
hypodermically injecting the composites into rats and
measuring the radioactivity of urine excretion at fixed
intervals of time. A control experiment performed by
injecting subcutaneously a solution of tritiated cyclazocine into rats equal to an average daily dose released by composite, showed that urinary excretion of
radioactivity is a useful measure for estimating the
cyclazocine released. A total recovery of 72% of the
dose administered was obtained. In the supposition
that the remaining 28% consisted of material released
through other ways and of experimental errors, the
values of the in vivo tests determined in urine with

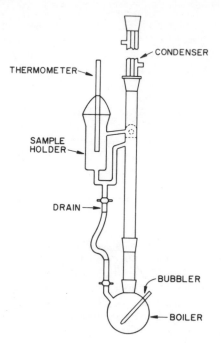

Figure 2.   Raab Extractor.

poly(lactic acid) (PLA) composites have been corrected
by this factor and are expressed as percent of the maximum dose released.

In control experiments performed as above using
naltrexone, a recovery of 30% of the administered dose
was obtained and consequently the values have been
corrected by this factor and are expressed as percent
of the maximum dose released. The cumulative amounts
of naloxone released are expressed as percent of dose
implanted for want of better evidence at this time.

In experiments in vitro, the delivery rates were
determined by extracting samples of the antagonist-
polymer composites with tepid water (29°±3) in a modified
Raab extractor (Figure 2) and measuring the radioactivity
of the extracted aqueous solution at fixed intervals of
time.

The physiological response in dogs was determined by
measuring the flexor reflex, the skin twitch reflex and
the pupillary diameter after injecting cyclazocine and
naltrexone composites with PLA and challenging with
morphine.

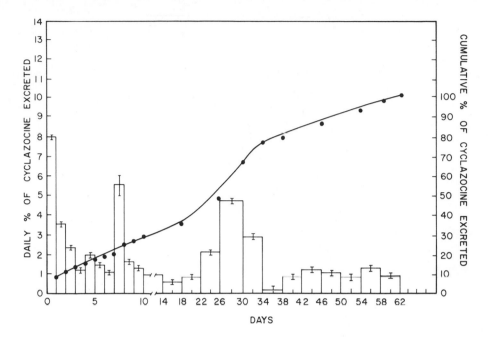

Figure 3.   Daily amounts of cyclazocine released from
composites with polyethylene in film form
on the left ordinate, and cumulative amounts
on the right ordinate, expressed as % of
implanted dose. Each point represents the
mean observation on three rats±S.E.

III.   RESULTS AND DISCUSSION

Composites in Film Form

Early experiments[5-7] with films of cyclazocine-
polyethylene composites implanted into rats indicated
the feasibility of the delivery system under investigation. The time at which one half of the implanted dose
had been released ($t_{\frac{1}{2}}$) was 27 days (Figure 3). The
average daily release was about 1%, after reaching higher
rates during the first week after implantation. Surprisingly, a significantly increased release was observed
between days 22 and 34.

Polyethylene has the disadvantage of requiring surgical removal of the polymeric matrix after the antagonist
has been delivered. To circumvent this problem, biodegradable poly(lactic acid) (PLA) was used in place of

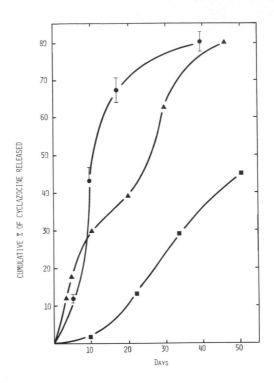

Figure 4.   Release of cyclazocine from polymeric films.
Each point in the in vivo experiments represents the mean observation on three
animals±S.E. ▲, polyethylene composites in
in vivo experiments (results expressed as %
of dose implanted); ●, PLA composites in in
viva experiments (results expressed as % of
maximum dose released); ■, PLA composites in
in vitro experiments.

polyethylene.[8] Sixty-two days after the implantation,
the polymeric matrix had practically disappeared, and
only tiny white specks remained at the implantation site.

     The in vivo release rate of cyclazocine from compo-
sites in film form with PLA is comparable to that
observed from composites with polyethylene, within
experimental errors (Figure 4). On the other hand, in
in vitro experiments cyclazocine is delivered from PLA
at a much slower rate than in vivo (Figure 4). Poor
correlation between in vivo and in vitro results has
been previously reported.[9-10]

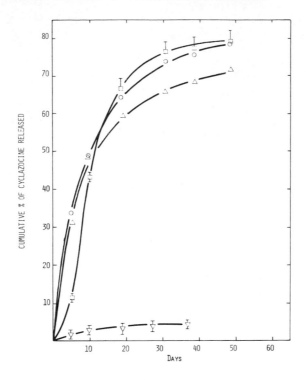

Figure 5.   Cumulative amounts of cyclazocine released
from composites of PLA in film form implanted
in rats, expressed as % of maximum dose released.   Each point represents the mean
observation on 3-4 animals±S.E.   The S.E.'s
for samples C and D are similar to that of
Sample B.   Molecular weights: ⊔, B, 70,000;
○, C, 45,000; and △, D, 60,000. ▽, E,
enveloped composite.

      Experiments in vivo with composites in film form
containing cyclazocine and PLA of molecular weights
varying from 45,000 to 70,000 showed that the release
rate of the antagonist is not very sensitive to variations in the molecular weight of the polymer (Figure 5).
The time at which half of the maximum dose had been delivered ($t_{1/2}$) was 13.0, 11.5, and 11.0 days for composites with PLA of molecular weights 70,000, 60,000,
and 45,000 respectively.[11]   The daily amount of cyclazocine excreted after reaching a maximum during the
first 3-5 days (Figure 6) decreased rapidly in the

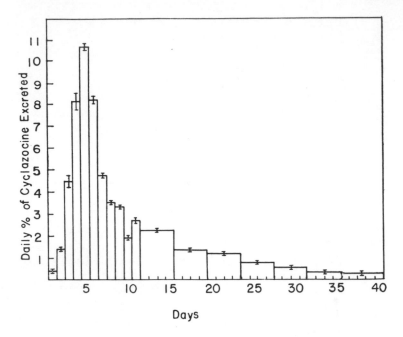

Figure 6.   Daily amounts of cyclazocine excreted, ex-
            pressed as % of the maximum dose released.
            Each point represents the mean observation
            on 9 animals±S.E. (Average of the results
            obtained in the experiments in vivo with
            samples B, C, and D.)

following 4 days, then remained relatively constant for
the duration of the tests at an average rate of 300
µg/kg/day. On a comparative basis this is approximately
10 times the human dose.

    Visual examination of the insertion area of the
sacrificed animals indicated that as expected the molecular weight of the polymer in the composites exerted a
significant influence on the rate of biodegradability,
with the lower molecular weight polymer being metabolized
faster.

    Delivery rates from films of composites sealed in
envelopes of pure polymer were also investigated. It
was thought that enveloping the composite would reduce
the initial delivery rate of cyclazocine. Experiments
were performed by enveloping a 6.2 cm^2 film of cyclazocine-PLA composite in a PLA film containing no cyclazocine, heat sealing the edges of the obtained envelope,
implanting the envelope into rats, and measuring the

excreted cyclazocine. An average total release of only
3.6% of cyclazocine in a 37 day interval was found
(Figure 5, sample E). In contrast, a 50% total release
of cyclazocine in 11 days was obtained from a non-
enveloped composite of the same composition (Figure 5,
sample C). These results indicate that the initial
delivery of the drug could be considerably reduced by
enveloping the composite and that a constant release of
cyclazocine can be obtained over a period of more than
a month.

Composites in Particle Form

A better delivery system for narcotic antagonists
would be small particles of composite hypodermically injected as a suspension into tissue instead of a surgically implanted film. Preliminary experiments performed
by injecting suspensions of small particles into rats of
cyclazocine-PLA composites in an aqueous solution of
carboxymethylcellulose showed the feasibility of this
system. The cumulative amount of cyclazocine excreted
within 54 days was 29% of the maximum dose released.
The time at which one quarter of the maximum dose had
been released ($t_{\frac{1}{4}}$) was 45 days (Figure 7). The daily
release (Figure 8) was approximately 0.5%, after a
slightly higher rate, about 2%, during the first 2 days
after injection.

When these particles were implanted surgically in
rats instead of injected as suspensions, no noticeable
difference in the release rates of cyclazocine was observed (Figure 7). Within 54 days 33% of the dose was
released in the implantation tests and 29% in the injection tests.

Comparison of these results obtained from particles
with those obtained from films (Figure 5, sample C),
shows that the in vivo release of cyclazocine from film
is at a surprisingly faster rate than from particles.
However, this is not inconsistent if consideration is
given to the fact that, after sacrificing the rats, a
larger amount of fluid was observed in the compartments
around the film than around the particles. Many factors
are involved in this inflammatory process. Films may
have produced a larger irritation than the particles,
possibly causing an increase in temperature surrounding
the composite, or a variation in the chemical composition of the body fluid or even in the mechanism by which

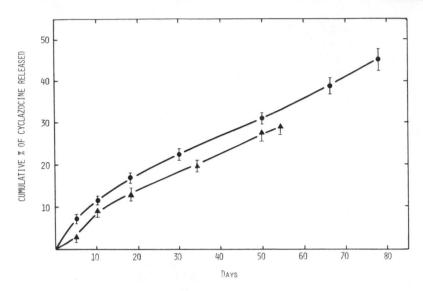

Figure 7.   In vivo release of cyclazocine from particles
            (falling within sieves Nos. 25/35 implanted
            (curve ●) and injected (curve ▲) into rats,
            expressed as % of maximum dose released.   Each
            point represents the mean observation on 2-4
            animals±S.E.

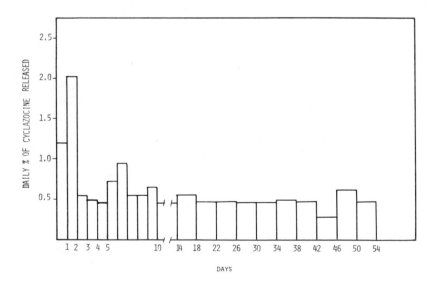

Figure 8.   In vivo daily release of cyclazocine from
            composites in particle form, expressed as %
            of maximum dose released.   Each point repre-
            sents the mean observation on 3 animals±S.E.

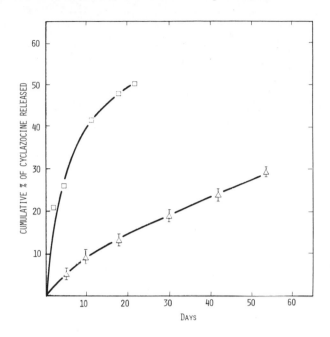

Figure 9. Cumulative amounts of cyclacozine released
from composites as small particles. □, in
vitro; △, in vivo (injected). Results
expressed as % of maximum dose released.
Each point represents the mean observation
on 3 animals±S.E.

the drug is transported. It is known that these variations accelerate the release rate of drugs.[12]

The in vitro delivery rate of cyclazocine from particles is faster than in vivo (Figure 9), as might be
expected due to the large excess of extractant present
in the in vitro tests.

From further investigation with composites in particle form, the in vivo and in vitro release rates of
naloxone and naltrexone were determined in comparison
with that of cyclazocine. The in vivo release rates
follow the order: naltrexone >cyclazocine >naloxone.
The cumulative amounts of naltrexone and cyclazocine
delivered in a 60 day period were, respectively, 68%
and 38% of the maximum dose released (Figure 10). In
the case of naloxone, 26% of the dose implanted was released during the same period (Figure 11). Parallel

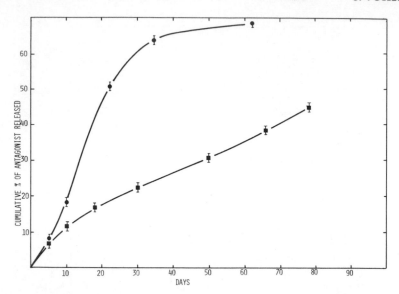

Figure 10.   In vivo release of cyclazocine (■) and
             naltrexone (●) from composites in particles
             falling within sieves No. 25/35.   Results
             expressed as % of maximum dose released.
             Each point represents the mean observation
             on 4 animals±S.E.

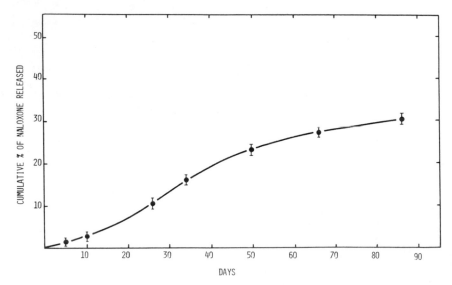

Figure 11.   In vivo release of naloxone from composites
             in particles falling between sieves Nos.
             25/35, expressed as % of the dose implanted.
             Each point represents the mean observation
             on 4 animals±S.E.

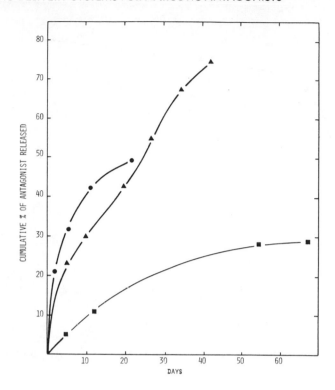

Figure 12.   In vitro release of cyclazocine (●), naloxone (■), and naltrexone (▲) from composi-
tions in particles falling between sieves
Nos. 25/35.

experiments in vitro showed that the delivery rates of
cyclazocine and naltrexone are considerably faster than
in vivo, whereas that of naloxone is surprisingly similar to that found in vivo, within experimental error
(Figure 12).   It appears from these tests that the in
vitro release of cyclazocine and naltrexone may be
different from that of naloxone. This behavior could
be due to differences in the physical make-up of the
composites, caused by the different melting points and
solubilities of these drugs in the polymer.

A structurally related antagonist, ℓ-BC-2605, is at
present under investigation. In experiments in vitro
the cumulative amount of ℓ-BC-2605 released in a 79 day
period was 63.7% of the dose. The release rate is
shown in Figure 13.

The encouraging results obtained with composites in
particle form led to the investigation of the influence

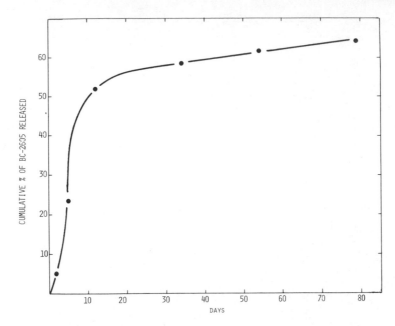

Figure 13. In vitro release of ℓ-BC-2605 from composites
            in PLA (particles falling between sieves
            Nos. 25/35).

of particle size on the rate of release. In experiments
in vitro and in vivo with naloxone composites, it was
found that the particle size of the composites, within
sieves Nos. 25/35 and 40/60 (0.71/0.50 and 0.42/0.25 mm)
shows only a moderate influence on the release rates of
the antagonist (Figure 14). Similar results have been
obtained with cyclazocine.

     Suspensions of cyclazocine-PLA composites in CM-
cellulose 7LS, when injected into dogs, produced a
blocking action lasting 8 days. This drug appears to
be more potent than morphine in producing depression of
the flexor reflex. Results obtained with naltrexone-
PLA composites showed blocking action toward morphine
for about 35 days in dogs.[13]

     Injection of suspensions of cyclazocine-PLA compo-
sites in CM-cellulose 7LS into mice produced during the
first 24 hours a 79% effective blocking action, which
decreased to 61% for the following seven days.[14]

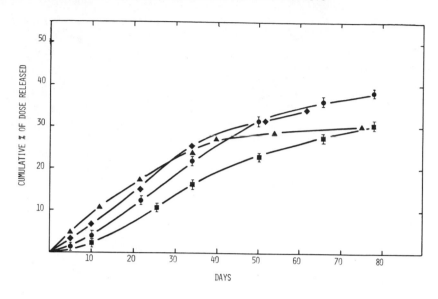

Figure 14.   Influence of particle size of composites on
             release rates of naloxone. Results of ex-
             periments *in vivo* expressed as percent of
             implanted dose. Each point represents the
             mean observation on 2-4 rats±S.E.

Symbol	Particles size falling between sieves Nos.	Experimental conditions
●	40/60 (0.42/0.25 mm)	*in vivo*
■	25/35 (0.71/0.50 mm)	*in vivo*
◆	40/60 (0.42/0.25 mm)	*in vitro*
▲	25/35 (0.71/0.50 mm)	*in vitro*

Migration Mechanism

     Two approaches have been investigated to describe
mathematically the migration of a drug through a polymer
matrix, shaped as films, pellets or cylinders. One makes
use of the classical Fick's laws of diffusion. In this
derivation, it is assumed that the drug is dissolved in
the medium in which it migrates and varies continuously
in concentration from the highest to the lowest values.

     The second approach, which modifies Fick's law, is
based on the assumption that the drug is scattered
through the polymer as small particles, with only a

minute fraction dissolved. These particles, which may
be considered as pockets or reservoirs of drug, diffuse
across the inside of the pockets, so that the walls of
the pockets are always saturated with drug as long as
any undissolved drug is present. During the migration
the drug escapes first from the pockets nearest the
exposed surfaces of the composite and tends to leave
the pockets in the interior of the composite only when
the pockets "ahead" of them have been emptied. Thus,
there will be a front or envelope of actively dischar-
ging pockets, which gradually recedes from the face of
the composite, for example a film, and disappears at
the mid-plane of the film. A similar approach has been
developed simultaneously.[3]

   Both mechanisms lead to results which can be expressed mathematically and plotted as delivery rate _vs_
time.[5]

REFERENCES

1.   T. Higuchi, _J. Pharm. Sci._, _50_, 874 (1961).

2.   T. Higuchi, _ibid._, _52_, 1145 (1963).

3.   T. J. Roseman and W. I. Higuchi, _ibid._, _59_,
     353 (1970) and T. J. Roseman, _ibid._, _61_, 46 (1972).

4.   a) B. Farhadieh, S. Borodkin and J. D. Buddenhagen,
     J. Pharm. Sci., _60_, 209 and 212 (1971).

     b) C. L. Levesque, U. S. Pat. 2,987,445 (1961).

5.   S. Yolles, J. E. Eldridge and J. H. R. Woodland,
     Polymer News, _1_, No. 4/5, 9 (1970).

6.   D. A. Blake, S. Yolles, M. Helrich, H. F. Cascorbi,
     and M. J. Eagan, "Release of Cyclazocine from Sub-
     cutaneously Implanted Polymeric Matrices", Abstract,
     Academy of Pharmaceutical Sciences, San Francisco,
     March 30, 1971.

7.   S. Yolles, "Development of a Long-Acting Dosage
     Form for Narcotic Antagonists", 13th National Medic-
     inal Chemistry Symposium, The University of Iowa,
     Iowa City, Iowa, June 18-22, 1972.

8.   R. K. Kulkarni, K. C. Pani, C. Newman, and F. Leonard, (Walter Reed Army Med. Center, Washington, D. C.) AD 636716. Avail. CFSTI, 15 pp. (1966).

9.   Y. C. Martin and C. Hansch, J. Med. Chem., 14, 777 (1971).

10. T. George, C. L. Kaul, R. D. Gremal, and D. V. Mehta, J. Med. Chem., 14, 909 (1971).

11. J. H. R. Woodland, S. Yolles, D. A. Blake, M. Helrich, and F. J. Meyer, J. Med. Chem., in press.

12. H. Lapidus and N. G. Lordi, J. Pharm. Sci., 57, 1292 (1968).

13. W. R. Martin and V. L. Sandquist, Paper presented at the 34th Annual Scientific Meeting of the Committee on Problems on Drug Dependence, sponsored by NRC and NAC, at the University of Michigan, Ann Arbor, Mi. May, 1972.

14. L. Harris and W. Dewey, Personal Communication, 1972.

CONTROLLED-RELEASE PESTICIDES: CONCEPTS AND REALIZATION

Amar Nath Neogi* and G. Graham Allan

University of Washington

Seattle, Washington 98195

I.   INTRODUCTION

Pesticides are agents that control plant and animal
life disadvantageous to man and his domestic animals.
Annual losses due to pests in any country are enormous,
and in the United States alone have been estimated to be
more than \$20 billion.[1-3] Pesticides for the control,
suppression, or destruction of plant or animal pests
thus play a vital role in our day-to-day life, both
economic and esthetic. Although these biologically
active compounds have been very effective in selectively
suppressing undesirable weeds and insects, thereby
tremendously increasing productive capacity of food
grains and dairy products[4] and irradicating many diseases
caused by insect vectors, there has been achieved very
little control over the persistence of activity of these
materials.

Very long-life pesticides (such as DDT) have been
undesirable because their residues enter the food chain.
On the other hand, pesticides with short lives have been
ineffective in controlling pests for a prolonged period.
The effective lives of both the durable and the ephemeral
pesticides are shortened by washing away by rain, by removal by evaporation, or by rapid biodegradation into
inactive components. Furthermore, such pesticides, after

---

*Present address: E. I. du Pont de Nemours & Co. (Inc.),
 Textile Fibers Department, Kinston, North Carolina 28501.

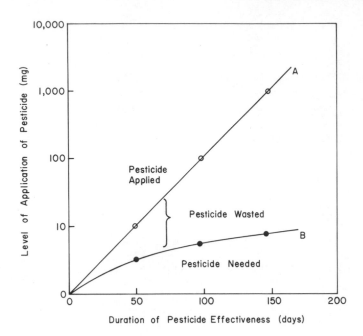

Figure 1.   Comparative duration of pesticide effective-
             ness for practical and ideal application
             levels.

application, may be leached out into subsoil, where breakdown is less rapid, and then into underground water
sources and possibly to streams and lakes with subsequent
damage to aquatic and wild life.[5-7]

     To compensate for losses, these biocides are commonly
applied in amounts grossly in excess of that theoreti-
cally expected to control the particular pest for a long
period.

     The reason behind such wasteful procedures is de-
picted graphically in Figure 1, which shows three levels
of application of a pesticide with a half-life of 15 days.
If the dissipation rate follows first order, then application of the pesticide just above the minimum level
necessary (say 1 mg) to control the pest would afford
protection for about a day. To achieve protection for
50 days, the level of conventional application would
have to increase tenfold, but only a third of the pesticide would be used for control of the target organism.

For double and triple this period of effectiveness, the levels of pesticide application must be multiplied by a hundred and a thousand, respectively.

On the other hand, if the pesticide could be maintained at the minimum required level (1 mg) by continuous supply to restore the fraction dissipated, then one can write for optimum performance:

$$\frac{dS}{dt} = \frac{dL}{dt} \tag{1}$$

rate of   rate of
supply   loss

Since the dissipation is assumed to be first-order,

$$\frac{dL}{dt} = k_L CV = k_L W \tag{2}$$

where k_L is the rate constant of pesticide loss obtained from the half-life of the biocide, and C is the concentration of the pesticide in volume V of the medium. Therefore:

$$\frac{dS}{dt} = k_L CV \tag{3}$$

and

$$dS = k_L W dt \tag{4}$$

where W is the weight of the pesticide in volume V. Since the minimum effective level of application is known (W = 1 mg), the incremental supply (dS) of the active ingredient is readily calculable.

Curve B of Figure 1 shows the amount needed to maintain the minimum effective level. The area between Curves A and B on the logarithmic scale represents the fraction of pesticide consumed without serving any useful purpose and points out clearly how much room exists for improvement in application techniques. Thus the total amounts needed for 50, 100, and 150 days of pest control are 3.3, 5.6, and 7.9 mg if the biocide is continuously replenished by a controlled-release mechanism, as contrasted to 10, 100, and 1000 mg by conventional application.

Obviously the efficacy of the pesticides already in use can be substantially increased in terms of their

duration of effectiveness, and the waste of these costly
chemicals, which may become the later cause of ecological crisis, can be reduced, by designing a system to
release these biologically active substances at a controlled rate - a rate high enough to be effective after
minimal losses from leaching by rain, removal by evaporation, and degradation. Any pesticide formulation which
can satisfy this criterion can be called a controlled-
release pesticide.

Various attempts have been made to control the release of pesticides from their formulations, and most
of these have been based on the concept of adsorbing the
pesticides on strong adsorbents like silica gel, mica,
and activated charcoal.[8-10] The strong forces of adsorption enable these carriers to slow the release through
an equilibrium favoring the adsorption site, but renewal
of the medium (e.g., by rain) can result in total release. The incomplete success of these formulations is
due to the nature of the release mechanism, which is
reversible.

Because many of these biologically active substances
are effective at very low concentrations, there exists
the possibility of controlling their release by use of
a polymer that contains the pesticide (a) dissolved,
encapsulated, or dispersed in it, so that release occurs
by diffusion of the pesticide through the polymer to the
surrounding medium, or (b) chemically bonded to the polymer by a hydrolyzable linkage, so that release occurs by
degradation of the linkage. Appropriately designed combinations should provide the required degree of protection for the desired length of time under a given set of
environmental conditions.

II.   ADVANTAGES OF CONTROLLED-RELEASE FORMULATIONS

As pointed out previously, controlled-release pesticides should allow much less pesticide to be used for
the same period of activity. In the conventional method
of control or suppression of pests, a disproportionately
larger amount of the active ingredient is used to achieve
a longer period of protection, and the amount of the
material wasted by leaching, evaporation, and degradation
is excessive. Since release under controlled conditions
would at all times provide just enough pesticide to offer
protection, i.e., would distribute the pesticide more
evenly with time, a much smaller amount would be needed

to offer the same period of activity. If a pesticide is chemically combined or dissolved or encapsulated in a polymeric material, its application to soil or any other medium would result in release of the active ingredient by hydrolysis or diffusion at a controlled rate; therefore the loss of the active ingredient by degradation, evaporation, or leaching would be minimized. Application of such combinations would therefore result in more efficient use of the active ingredients per unit weight and would result in a much longer period of protection for the same amount, than if applied by conventional method. Since the biocide would be encased in a polymeric cage, it would be less susceptible to attack by bacteria or fungi. Combinations designed to offer prolonged protection would thereby eliminate the cost of repeated and over applications.

Many of the newer pesticides, which are readily biodegradable and therefore desirable, are highly toxic. The organophosphates are especially potent, and efficient respiratory protective devices are recommended for persons handling these insecticides. Because of their mobility in water and air, their application also is a source of danger to nontarget organisms like aquatic and wild life. If these materials were chemically contained within a polymer, they should become much less toxic, since all of the active ingredient would not be released at one time. Moreover, the polymeric combination of pesticides, being solid and less toxic, could be easily handled and transported from one place to another. Furthermore they could be processed and distributed by conventional machinery.

The large amounts of pesticides applied to achieve protection for a long time sometimes cause phytotoxicity. Since a controlled-release formulation would not release the active ingredients all at once, this problem should not arise. Moreover, a combination of pesticide with polymer should minimize errors of measuring and diluting liquid concentrates. A polymer combination of a pesticide in the solid form should be easily deposited precisely where it will perform most efficiently, and thus minimize waste. Because the actual amount of pesticide needed for a biological response is small, the material released under controlled conditions would be substantially absorbed by the host or trapped and degraded in the soil. By eliminating the wide-spread distribution of large amounts of pesticides, saturation of the ecological environment would be avoided, and the leaching

of pesticides by rain into waterways and subsoil should
be alleviated. Some rather stable pesticides or their
degradation products now find their way into potable
water supplies and can end up in humans through food
consumption, with the attendant possibility of health
problems in the long term.[11-13] If leaching could be
minimized, herbicides could be used more safely near
irrigation canals and near crops especially sensitive
to some of these agents.

      The excessive dissemination of pesticides into the
terrestrial and aquatic acosystems and the accumulation
of solid wastes of various types are both major environmental concerns. It may be possible to combine apparently negative features of both to provide a positive
solution for their simultaneous reduction.[14] The
prodigious amount of solid wastes, totalling about 165
million tons in the United States alone, consists pre-
dominantly of bark, sawdust, bagasse, and other cellu-
losic wastes, and leather, cannery, and other protein-
aceous wastes. If these could be chemically combined
with pesticides, e.g., herbicides, by hydrolyzable
linkages to gain controlled release, the cost of dis-
posing of the solid wastes (about $3 billion/yr) could
be reduced, and the reduction would add to the savings
afforded by controlled release in reducing waste of
chemicals and cost of application. What was a liability
could become an asset. Furthermore, the residue after
release of the pesticide could improve the quality of
the soil by reducing the amount of dust and increasing
the porosity.[15] Thus, the use of polymeric pesticides
integrates with other efforts to limit pesticide build-
up in the environment and develop short-lived pesticides.

                    III. PRIOR RESEARCH

      The use of polymers to control the release of biolog-
ically active ingredients and nutrients is a relatively
new concept, and only a few reports appear in recent
literature. One method[16] utilized a physical release
mechanism in which the pesticide was adsorbed on a
carrier and then coated with a urea-formaldehyde resin.
Insecticides have been mixed with polymers to obtain
biocidal formulations which have an extended life yet
provide an increase in the safety of otherwise toxic
compounds.[17] Another method[18] employs a poly(butyl
acrylate) latex with added O,O-dimethyl-O-(2,4,5-tri-
chlorophenyl) phosphorothioate. This modified latex

when sprayed on cattle is reported to prevent horsefly
infestation for three weeks. Protection has also been
achieved by feeding livestock the insecticide incorporated in a urea-formaldehyde or polyester resin.[19]

Chlorinated phenols have been incorporated into
alkyd resins as esters of tri- or tetracarboxylic acids
of benzene, and coatings of the resin are claimed to have
fungicidal properties.[20] Pentachlorophenyl acrylate, a
well known fungicide, has been homo- and copolymerized
with other monomers to result in polymers which are
fungicidal.[21]

Long-term control of barnacles on ships has been
achieved by coating the underwater surfaces with paints
containing the trimer of phenarsazine chloride or the
polyacrylate of tributyltin hydroxide.[22-23]

A recent patent[24] claims that alkyd resins with
chemically bonded herbicides have a longer effective
life than the herbicide alone. These are formed by incorporating a herbicide, such as Fenone (2,4-DEP),
which is tris(2,4-dichlorophenoxyethyl)phosphite, a
nonvolatile, water-insoluble liquid which breaks down
in moist soil releasing 2,4-dichlorophenoxyethanol,[25]
into the reaction mixture of phthalic anhydride or
humic acid and glycerol to form a hard friable resin.
The utilization of forest wastes and other low-cost
materials to produce sustained-release herbicides is
claimed in another patent.[26]

Pesticides embedded or encapsulated in polymeric
matrices constitute the basis of Shell Chemical Company's
well known No-Pest Strip®.[27] Recently the Pennwalt
Corporation obtained an experimental label from the
Environmental Protection Agency clearing the way for
large-scale field tests of a polyamide-encapsulated
methylparathion.[28]

These examples of the use of polymers either chemically or physically combined with the pesticide component indicate a great potential of achieving better
utilization of herbicides, insecticides, molluscicides,
rodenticides, plant-growth regulators, and the like.
However, realization of the potential will not be
approached until much basic information is obtained
from fundamental design studies.

IV. DESIGN AND DEVELOPMENT OF
CONTROLLED-RELEASE PESTICIDES

We, at the University of Washington, through studies
of the various ways of making controlled-release formulations and the effects of polymer properties on release
rates, have sought to place pest control on a sound quantitative and predictive basis, so that polymeric combinations can be designed to release active components at
desired rates for predetermined periods, possibly independent of minor changes in the surroundings.

In order to design a controlled-release formulation
of a biocide to offer protection for a predetermined
period, it is necessary to determine the variables which
affect the release rate.[29,30] The rate of release is
governed by the mechanism by which the active ingredient
is supplied to the medium, and therefore the pertinent
variables are different for different modes of release.
Controlled-release formulations can be classified on the
basis of release mechanisms into: (1) physical combinations, in which the pesticide is released from the polymer by a diffusion process: and (2) chemical combinations, in which the pesticide is released by a slow
degradation or cleavage of the pesticide-polymer linkage.
Let us now consider the design factors associated with
each.

Physical Combinations

Selection of Pesticide and Polymer. Two basic factors influencing the design of a controlled-release system are obviously the structure of the pesticide and the
structure of the polymeric matrix. The former is of
course determined by the particular plant or animal pest
and is usually substantially invariant. In contrast the
structure of the polymeric moiety of a combination can
be varied greatly. For reasons of convenience and eco-
nomics, it is preferable to select a matrix material
which is available commercially. Unfortunately, most
commercial polymers are unsuitable because they are in-
compatible with biocides. Surprisingly, however, substantially linear polyurethanes or polyamides are excellent solvents for almost every systemic biocide now used,
and within each class of polymeric materials are a large
number of members, such as nylons 4, 5, 6, 610, 66, 7, 9,
11, and 12, many of which are available commercially.
Because mixing a biocide with a molten polymer would be
the preferred method of incorporation, polymers of low

softening points are desired to prevent thermal degradation of the biologically active ingredient. Moreover,
polymers of high crystallinity should be avoided, since,
in a highly ordered matrix, the release of dissolved
material from the matrix can lead to its shrinkage and
fracture, which would alter the release rate.

The use of an elastic polymeric matrix of low softening point is therefore desirable. Since the high melting temperatures and crystallinity of nylons are
attributed to the presence of hydrogen bonds and a relatively high frequency of amide groups along the polymer
chain,[31-32] nylons of greater value for controlled release can be made by interposing a bulky unit to restrict hydrogen-bond formation and serve as an internal
plasticizer. The dimer of linoleic acid, which is a
commercially available relatively low-cost material,[33]
can function in this manner, and its condensation
polymer (I) with ethylenediamine has suitable solvent
and melt-flow characteristics.

$$\left[\text{NHCO(CH}_2)_8 \quad\quad \text{CH}_2\text{CH=CH(CH}_2)_7\text{CONHCH}_2\text{CH}_2\right]_n$$

$$-(\text{CH}_2)_4\text{CH}_3$$

$$(\text{CH}_2)_4\text{CH}_3$$

(I)

Rate of Pesticide Release.   The rate of release
of a biocide from a polymer-pesticide combination is
governed by Fick's law of diffusion.[22-32]   For an iso-
tropic system in rectangular cartesian co-ordinates,

$$\frac{\partial C}{\partial t} = \frac{\partial}{\partial x}\left(D\frac{\partial C}{\partial x}\right) + \frac{\partial}{\partial y}\left(D\frac{\partial C}{\partial y}\right) + \frac{\partial}{\partial z}\left(D\frac{\partial C}{\partial z}\right) \quad\quad (5)$$

where C is the concentration of the pesticide at a point
(x, y, z) in the polymer at an elapsed time t, and D is
the diffusivity of the pesticide.

The boundary conditions to which a particular combination is subjected depends on its particular application. A knowledge of the diffusion coefficient, D,

along with the boundary conditions would therefore allow
a prediction of release rate.

Determination of Diffusivity. When we consider the
diffusion in one dimension, Equation (5) reduces to

$$\frac{\partial C}{\partial t} = \frac{\partial}{\partial x}\left(D\frac{\partial C}{\partial x}\right) \tag{6}$$

where D, the diffusivity at point x, is dependent on C,
the concentration at point x.

For polymers, the concentration dependency is usually
given by[34,35]

$$D = D_o e^{sC} \tag{7}$$

where $D = D_o$ when $s = 0$ or $C = 0$, s being the nonideality coefficient.

Now the flux, dQ/dt, as defined by Fick's first law
of diffusion is

$$\frac{dQ}{dt} = -D_o\left(\frac{\partial C}{\partial x}\right)\Big|_{x=o} \tag{8}$$

For a semi-infinite medium with boundary conditions $C = 0$
at $x = 0$ and $C = C_o$ at $x = \infty$ at elapsed time, t, Boltzman
transformation of Equation (6) using $y = x/2(D_o t)^{\frac{1}{2}}$ and
subsequent rearrangement gives:

$$\frac{dQ}{dt} = -\frac{C_o}{2}\left(D_o t\right)^{\frac{1}{2}}\left(\frac{d\ C/C_o}{dy}\right)\Big|_{y=o} \tag{9}$$

Integration with respect to time gives the net amount
released:

$$Q_t = mt^{\frac{1}{2}} \tag{10}$$

$$\text{where}\qquad m = C_o D_o^{\frac{1}{2}}\left(\frac{d\ C/C_o}{dy}\right)\Big|_{y=o} \tag{11}$$

Thus, a plot of Q_t against $t^{\frac{1}{2}}$ should yield a straight
line of slope m, particularly for relatively small values
of time. It must be recognized that the components of m
are dependent on the values of C_o, D_o, and s.

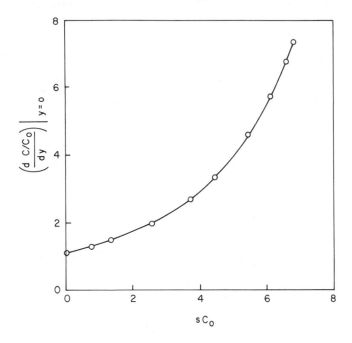

Figure 2.   Effect of nonideality constant s on the dimen-
             sionless concentration gradient at the surface.

Therefore, determination of the magnitude of m at two
values of C_O would permit the evaluation of s and D_O,
provided the dependency of $(d\ C/C_O)/(dy)|_{y=0}$ with sC_O is
known.   Figure 2, which was obtained by a computer solution of Equation (6), represents such relationship.[36]

Experimental plots of the rate of biocide release
against $t^{\frac{1}{2}}$ for two values of initial concentration (C)
would afford values of both D_O and s by a trial and
error technique.   Hence the rates of pesticide release
and the duration of protection can be predicted.

For experimental verification of this analysis, a
series of controlled-release biocide polymer combinations
were prepared and the release rates of the biocide were
determined from blocks of these combinations by exposing
one surface of the block to water.

The model pesticide selected was HMPT, a housefly
chemosterilant[37] which is infinitely soluble in water

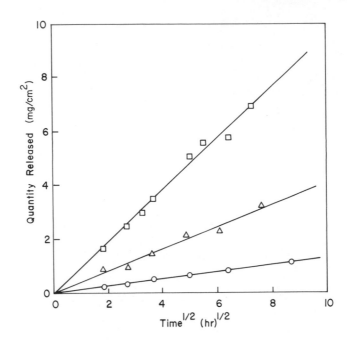

Figure 3. Total release of the pesticide per unit area
           from a semi-infinite polymer block as a func-
           tion of square-root of time. Polymer $\overline{M}_n$,
           15,000. C_o, $\square$, 21.48%; $\triangle$, 14.00%;
           $\bigcirc$, 6.90%.

Table I. Dependence of Diffusion Coefficient on
          Polymer Matrix Molecular Weight and
                Pesticide Concentration

Polymer Molecular Weight, $\overline{M}_n$	$D_o \times 10^{10}$ cm^2/sec	s
2000	20.71	17.80
6000	7.90	19.15
9800	5.93	20.28
15000	4.67	20.93

and thermally stable (b.p. 253°). The polymers used were
a series of polyamides with number-average molecular
weights ($\overline{M}_n$) of 2000 to 15,000 prepared from ethylene
diamine and dilinoleic acid. Plots of the pesticide released against square root of elapsed time were straight
lines as shown in Figure 3. From the slopes of the
lines, the values of D_o and s were calculated and are
presented in Table I for different molecular weights of
polymers.

The change in diffusivity with molecular weight is
particularly noteworthy and is due to the presence of
a larger amount of oligomers in the lower-molecular-
weight matrix than in higher ones.

The excellent agreement of the experimental data with
the theoretical prediction is evidence that rational de-
signs for physical forms of controlled-release biocides
can be developed.

Chemical Combinations

As opposed to the physical combinations of active
ingredients dissolved in polymers, chemical combinations
have the pesticide firmly attached to the polymeric substrate by a definite identifiable chemical bond and can
therefore be obtained only if the pesticide has at least
one reactive functional moiety. The attachment can take
any one of the several forms illustrated in Figure 4.
The simplest example is the attachment of the biocide as
a pendant substituent[38] to a natural or synthetic water-
soluble or insoluble polymer having a replaceable hydrogen as shown in Equation (12):

$$\text{Polymer-L-H} + \text{RCOOH} \underset{\text{environment}}{\overset{\text{synthesis}}{\rightleftharpoons}} \text{Polymer-L-COR} \quad (12)$$

(L = N, 0, or S)

Combinations of this type can be readily synthesized by
conventional procedures. Where the pesticide cannot be
directly attached to the polymer to form a suitable bond,
a bridging entity may be interposed. An example of this
would be the linkage of a pesticide amine to a poly-
saccharide substrate by means of a dianhydride or di-
urethane bridge. Alternatively the pesticide may be
initially converted to a polymerizable derivative, e.g.,
vinyl 2-methyl-4-chlorophenoxyacetate, which is then

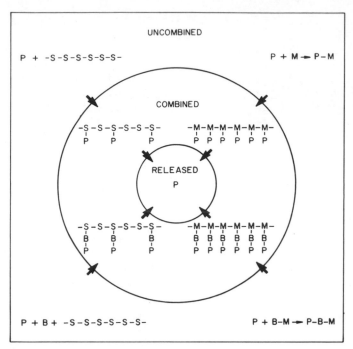

Figure 4.   Routes to synthesis of controlled-release
             chemical combinations.

homo- or copolymerized to give a wholly synthetic pesticide-polymer combination as illustrated in Figure 4.

    Selection of Substrate.   Obviously the rate of re-
lease of the active ingredient and consequent efficacy
and duration would depend on the properties of the macro-
molecule and its surrounding medium.   The characteristics
of the polymeric biocide would largely be derived from:
(1) the nature of pesticide-polymer bonds; (2) the chemical characteristics of the monomers and co-monomers; and
(3) the dimension and structure of the polymer molecule
as governed by degree of polymerization, degree of crosslinking, and the stereochemistry.

    The rate of hydrolysis and hence the rate of release
depends on the strength and chemical nature of the polymer-pesticide bond.   For example, an anhydride linkage
is more susceptible than an ester linkage to alkaline
hydrolysis.   The rate of hydrolysis of a linkage is also
dependent on the groups surrounding it.   Hydrophobic

groups thus offer protection against hydrolysis. For
example, a copolymer of acrylic acid and p-nitrophenyl
acrylate hydrolyzes much faster than the homopolymer of
the latter.[41] This is further supported by the work of
Davies, 'et al.[42-43] who determined the rate of saponifi-
cation of various copolymers of vinyl esters.

Dimension, structure, and stereochemistry also play
a role in the rate of release by hindering the approach
to a particular bond in question. Thus a highly crosslinked polymer is much less susceptible to hydrolysis
compared to an uncrosslinked one, and a stereoregular
or crystalline polymer is less susceptible than an amorphous or atactic polymer. Hence it is necessary to know
the characteristics of the polymer which in combination
with pesticide would offer protection and maintain the
advantages of a controlled-release pesticide. Previous
attempts[44] to use controlled-release formulations of
some phenoxy-acid herbicides have failed possibly because an inappropriate polymer was chosen. To determine
the nature of an acceptable polymer, we synthesized a
series of herbicide-polymer compounds and evaluated them
for their biological activity. The pesticides and
monomers chosen and the polymers synthesized are shown
in Tables II and III which also include their biological
effectiveness. Their effectiveness was measured by their
ability to prevent the germination of lettuce seeds. The
positive sign (+) indicates effectiveness while the zero
sign (0) indicates absence of biological activity.

Table IV gives the time periods for which various
amounts of these combinations offer protection compared
with those of the pesticides alone.

It is apparent from these tables that for a polymer-
pesticide combination to be effective as a sustained-release or controlled-release pesticide, the polymer must
have some hydrophilic group to enhance the degradation
rate. The number of these groups needed would depend on
the characteristics of the medium and the nature of the
linkage. An anhydride linkage would need the least percentage of hydrophilic groups. The frequency of such
groups would affect the period of activity as shown by
the duration of effectiveness of the copolymers of 2,3,5-
trichloro-4-pyridyl methacrylate and acrylic acid. As
shown in Table IV, a higher percentage of acrylic acid
offers protection for less time than that with a lower
one, because large numbers of $-CO_2H$ groups on the chain
make the surrounding ester linkages more susceptible to

Table II. Biological Effectiveness of Polymeric Pesticides

Pesticide P-OH	Pesticide Monomer	Polymer	Intrinsic Viscosity	Biological Activity
CH₃ — ring (OCH₂COOH, Cl)	P-OCH=CH₂	homopolymer of vinyl ester	0.14	0
CH₃ — ring (OCH₂COOH, Cl)	P-OCH=CH₂	copolymer of vinyl ester and acrylic acid	0.10	+
CH₃ — ring (OCH₂COOH, Cl)	P-OCH₂CHCH₂ (O)	homopolymer of glycidyl ester	0.05	+
ring (OH, Cl, Cl, Cl, Cl)	P-OCOC(CH₃)=CH₂	homopolymer of methacrylic ester	0.08	0
ring (OH, Cl, Cl, Cl, N)	P-OCOC(CH₃)=CH₂	homopolymer of methacrylic ester	0.15	0
ring (OH, Cl, Cl, Cl, N)	P-OCOC(CH₃)=CH₂	copolymer of methacrylic ester and acrylic acid	0.15	+

Table III. Biological Effectiveness of Controlled-Release Combinations of Pesticide and Polymer

Pesticide	Polymer	Pesticide Content, %	Biological Activity
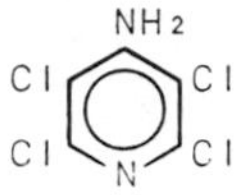	Dowex A-1 aluminum chelate	10.5	0
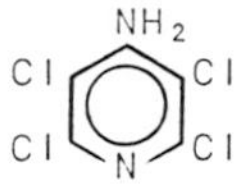	Dowex A-1 iron chelate	8.3	+
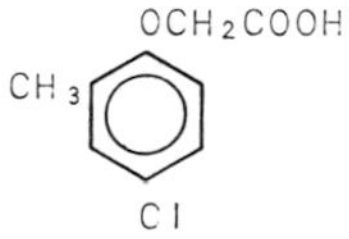	poly(vinyl alcohol)	56.1	+
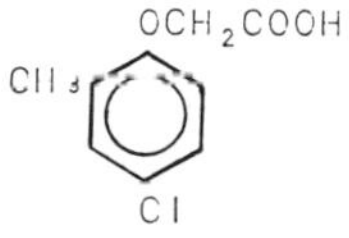	kraft lignin	38.5	+
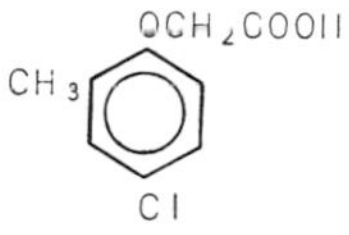	bark	51.1	+
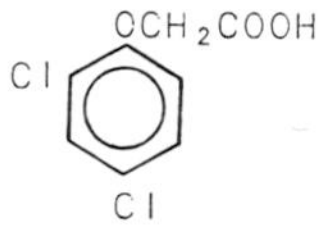	α-cellulose	73.2	+

Table IV. Period of Protection Offered by Various Controlled-Release Combinations

Pesticide	Form	Amount of Pesticide Applied, mg	Period of Protection, Days
2-methyl-4-chlorophenoxyacetic acid	control	100	45
	vinyl ester of pesticide copolymerized with acrylic acid	100	60
	pesticide combined with kraft lignin	100	115
	pesticide combined with bark	100	100
	control	250	60
	pesticide combined with poly(vinyl alcohol)	225	95
2,3,5-trichloro-4-hydroxypyridine	control	100	20
	95.2/4.8 copolymer of methacrylic ester and acrylic acid	100	70
	57.9/42.1 copolymer of methacrylic ester and acrylic acid	100	35
4-amino-3,5,6-trichloropicolinic acid	control	50	30
	chelate polymer of Dowex A-1 resin	50	80

attack and also serve as catalysts for hydrolysis of the neighboring ester linkages. Table IV is further evidence that a pesticide-polymer combination offers much longer protection compared to the pesticide itself for an equivalent amount of pesticide.

Rate of Release. After establishing the essential features needed for a polymer containing the pesticide to release effectively, it is necessary to determine the effective persistence of activity of these polymers and hence the rates of release. The persistence of activity of a particular formulation is determined by a bioassay technique to measure the time at which the release of the pesticide fails to make up the loss. The rate at this time is denoted by R_c.

In a medium saturated with water, the rate of hydrolysis for heterogeneous surface reaction can be written for water-insoluble polymers

$$-\rho n 4 \pi r^2 \frac{dr}{dt} = k n 4 \pi r^2 C_o \qquad (13)$$

where n is the number of particles of average radius r at time t, k is the rate constant, ρ is the density, and C_o is the concentration of P-polymer linkages. C_o is a constant for a particular polymer because as one biocide molecule escapes from the surface, the water finds another combined P behind. The following equations apply:

$$-\rho \frac{dr}{dt} = k C_o \qquad (14)$$

$$r_o - r = \frac{k}{\rho} C_o t \qquad (15)$$

$$R_c = k n 4 \pi r_o^2 C_o = k n 4 \pi \left(r_o - \frac{k}{\rho} C_o t c \right)^2 C_o \qquad (16)$$

$$r_o - \frac{k}{\rho} C_o t_c = \left(\frac{R_c}{k n 4 \pi C_o} \right)^{\frac{1}{2}} \qquad (17)$$

Therefore

$$t_c = \frac{\rho r_o}{k C_o} - \left(\frac{R_c \rho^2}{n k^3 4 \pi C_o^3} \right)^{\frac{1}{2}} \qquad (18)$$

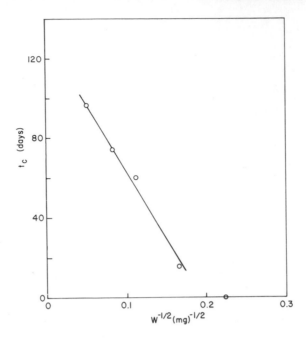

Figure 5.   The period of protection (t_c) offered by
             various amounts (W) of poly(vinyl alcohol)-
             2-methyl-4-chlorophenoxyacetic acid combina-
             tion.

Since n is proportional to the amount of combination W,
we can write

$$t_c = K_1 - K_2 W^{-\frac{1}{2}} \qquad (19)$$

$$K_1 = \frac{\rho r_o}{k C_o} \quad \text{and} \quad K_2 = \left(\frac{R_c \rho^3 r_o^3}{3 k^3 C_o^3} \right)^{\frac{1}{2}}$$

     The persistence time plotted against $W^{-\frac{1}{2}}$ should
accordingly yield a straight line with the slope K_2 and
intercept K_1.

     The validity of this equation was demonstrated by
measuring the persistence of herbicidal activity exhibited by a polymer synthesized by the partial acylation
(56.1%) of poly(vinyl alcohol) with 2-methyl-4-chloro-
phenoxyacetyl chloride (Figure 5).

When the hydrolyzed polymer is insoluble (<u>e.g.</u>, cellulose or lignin), the rate of cleavage can be written as

$$-\frac{dC}{dt} = k_2 C \tag{20}$$

$$-\frac{dC}{C} = k_2 dt \tag{21}$$

$$\ln C_o/C = k_2 t \tag{22}$$

where C is the concentration of pesticide per unit weight at time t, and k_2 is the degradation rate constant.

Now
$$R_c = k_2 W C_o e^{-k_2 t_c} \tag{23}$$

or
$$t_c = \frac{1}{k_2} \log W - \frac{1}{k_2} \log \frac{R_c}{k_2} \tag{24}$$

Equation (24) predicts that a plot of t_c against log W will be a straight line.

Experimental confirmation of the usefulness of Equation (23) in the design of controlled release pesticide-polymer combinations is provided by the release of herbicide acids from the esters of cellulose and lignin (Figure 6).

VI.   APPLICATIONS OF CONTROLLED-RELEASE PESTICIDES

The number of applications that can be visualized for controlled-release combinations is immense. Moreover, the concept is applicable to the release of other biologically active substances. In the University of Washington program, the major effect has been directed toward field testing the theories developed, in a forestry context, both in tropical and temperate regions. As for example, reforestration with productive conifers is usually retarded by the rapid invasion of competitive vegetation. Although this problem is well recognized, its control by herbicide is not simple. A herbicide is required which is selectively toxic to the unwanted brush with a period of protection on the order of several years. The chlorophenoxy butyric acids[45] are the most

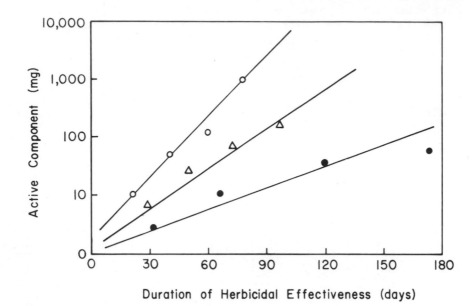

Figure 6.   Relationship of duration of herbicidal
             effectiveness to level of application for
             2,4-dichlorophenoxyacetic acid (2,4-D)
             chemically combined with water-insoluble
             polymers. O, 2,4-D alone; △, 19.7%
             2,4-D/Douglas fir bark chemical combina-
             tion; ●, 39% 2,4-D/kraft lignin chemical
             combination.

promising pesticides found in this regard. However,
these herbicides are readily oxidized in the soil by a
β-oxidase enzyme to the corresponding chlorophenoxy-
acetic acids which are toxic to the conifers. In this
case the controlled-release pesticide combination is
being utilized to perform a dual role:[46] it greatly
enhances the period of effectiveness through a single
application of the herbicide; and it reduces enzymatic
oxidation of the butyric acid herbicide to the corresponding acetic acid in the soil.

Field Tests

Ester combinations of 2,4-dichloro-phenoxybutyric
acid (2,4-DB) with bark were synthesized and their
selective toxicity was evaluated to western red alder
(Alnus rubra Bong.) in the presence of Douglas fir
(Pseudotsuga menziesii[Mirb]Franco) in the green house.

In Tables V, VI, and VII are presented the toxicological data which show that an application level of 10 g
effectively eliminates the unwanted vegetation without
damaging the conifers. A field evaluation is under way
to evaluate the practical feasibility of this approach
The field site near Sedro Woolley, Washington, covers
an area of 10,000 yards^2, containing about 800 Douglas-
fir seedlings. The seedlings were treated with the
controlled-release combinations containing 37% of
2,4-DB at four levels of application. After one growing
season, it was found that the height increase for the
treated seedlings was double that of the untreated seedlings and at the same time, the competitive vegetation
was reduced to one-third. To assess the effect of
climatic and soil conditions, field trials of similar
nature are underway in various parts of the country.
The suppression of vegetation by controlled-release
herbicides along railroads, fire breaks and power-line
right-of-ways is also being studied in a number of
field trials.

With increasing demand of the lumber industry, efforts are being made to cultivate commercially valuable
woods in the tropics. A typical acre of tropical forest
contains approximately 150 tree species and only one or
two of these are commercially useful. Planting efforts
to extend the number of Spanish cedar or mahogany in
these tropical American forests have been set back by
devastating attacks of a lepidopteran shootborer,
Hypsipyla grandela Zeller.[47-48] The larvae of this moth
find their way into stems of seedlings eventually causing crippling distortion or death. Protection by pesticides in conventional form is not economically feasible
because such applications last only two weeks under the
climatic conditions of heavy and frequent rains. Applications of controlled-release combinations could be
effective because such combinations can prolong the
period of effectiveness of the systemic insecticide in
one application by constantly replenishing the used or
decomposed biocide and at the same time reducing the
biocide loss by leaching or biodegradation. Evaluation

Table V.　Effect of Controlled-Release 2,4-DB-Bark Combinations on the Extent of Crown Kill in Douglas Fir and Western Red Alder Seedlings

Amount of Herbicide-Bark Combination Applied, g	Releasable Herbicide Content, %	Average Height, cm, of Transplanted Seedling at Time of Treatment		Extent of Crown Kill, %	
		Douglas Fir	W. Red Alder	Douglas Fir	W. Red Alder
10	50	25	37	0	100
55	50	26	38	100	100
100	50	25	38	100	100
10	37	26	38	0	100
55	37	24	37	100	100
100	37	25	38	100	100
10	31	30	46	0	75
55	31	32	47	75	100
100	31	31	45	100	100

Table VI. Effect of Controlled-Release Chemical Combinations of
2,4-DB on the Extent of Height Increase of Douglas Fir
and Western Red Alder After One Growing Season

| Amount of Herbicide-Bark Combination Applied, g | Releasable Herbicide Content, % | Height Increase, %, for | | | |
| | | Douglas Fir | | Western Red Alder | |
		Untreated	Treated	Untreated	Treated
10	50	55	54	80	0
10	37	54	56	78	0
10	31	49	50	68	16

Table VII. Effect of Controlled-Release Chemical Combinations of 2,4-DB on the Extent of Root Competition Around Douglas Fir and Western Red Alder Seedlings After One Growing Season

Amount of Herbicide-Bark Combination Applied, g	Releasable Herbicide Content, %	Vegetation Yield, g, Around			
		Douglas Fir		Western Red Alder	
		Untreated	Treated	Untreated	Treated
10	50	8	0	17	0
55	50	10	0	10	0
100	50	6	0	17	0
10	37	10	0	15	0.2
55	37	7	0	12	0
100	37	5	0	10	0
10	31	6	0.1	9	0.2
55	31	5	0	8	0
100	31	6	0	11	0

of preliminary controlled-release forms of readily biodegradable carbamate and organophosphates offer much
longer protection - over a year's protection has been
obtained in the best case[49] and thus the trees have been
protected from the massive attack potential of eight
pest generations. Combinations[50] have been designed to
extend this period to 5 years and are being evaluated in
Costa Rica, Puerto Rico and the Virgin Islands.

   The above two examples are the forerunners of the
new breed of pest control systems that will bring forth
ecological compatibility and simultaneously smooth the
inevitable transition from the old empirical broad spec-
trum use of chemicals to the more modern specific biological controls such as pheromones that are beginning
to emerge and will need to be dispensed in a controlled
fashion.

                        REFERENCES

1.   O. Johnson, N. Krog, J. L. Poland, Chemical Week,
     May 25 and June 1, 1963.

2.   Agr. Handbook, 291, U. S. Dept. Agr. (1965).

3.   A. Moseman, Natl. Res. Council, Publ. 1402, Washing-
     ton, D. C., 1966, p. 26.

4.   R. L. Metcalf, Encyclopedia of Chemical Technology,
     15, 2nd Ed. 908 (1968).

5.   M. B. Etteinger and D. J. Mount, Environ. Sci. Tech.,
     1, 203 (1967).

6.   P. H. Nicholson, Science, 158, (1967).

7.   N. A. Camrasni, Eau, 54, 579 (1967).

8.   J. W. Nemec and E. A. Nolan, U. S. Pat. 3,194,730
     (July 13, 1968).

9.   A. F. Caprio and W. Horback, U. S. Pat. 2,460,376
     (Feb. 1, 1949).

10. B. Wolfgang, U. S. Pat. 3,127,235 (March 31, 1964).

11.   "Bibliography of Organic Pesticide Predictions Hav-
      ing Relevance to Public Health and Water Pollution
      Problems". Project No. GL-WP-3 prepared for New
      York State Dept. of Health by the Syracuse Univer-
      sity Research Corp., May 1963.

12.   E. Hindin, M. J. Hatten, D. S. May, R. T. Skrinde,
      and G. H. Dustan, J. Am. Waterworks Assoc., 54,
      88 (1962).

13.   R. L. Woodward, J. Am. Waterworks Assoc., 52,
      1367 (1960).

14.   G. G. Allan, C. S. Chopra, A. N. Neogi, and R. M.
      Wilkins, Int. Pest. Control, Jan.-Feb. (1971).

15.   J. A. Krupenikow and N. I. Rogovskaya, Khim v.
      Sel'sk Khoz., 4 (6), 455 (1966).

16.   R. J. Geary, U. S. Pat. 3,074,845 (Jan. 22, 1963).

17.   R. J. Geary, U. S. Pat. 3,223,513 (Dec. 14, 1965).

18.   R. T. McFadden, R. R. Langer, and L. L. Wade, U. S.
      Pat. 3,212,967 (Oct. 19, 1965) and 3,228,830
      (January 11, 1966).

19.   J. E. Lloyd and J. G. Matthysse, Econ. Entomol.,
      59, 363 (1965).

20.   R. L. Broadhead, U. S. Pat. 3,179,608 (April, 1965).

21.   G. Faerber, Brit. Pat. 826,831 (Jan. 20, 1960).

22.   M. Nagahisa and K. Akagane, Chem. & Ind. (Japan),
      24, 127 (1967).

23.   R. Sano and K. Machihara, Color Material, Material
      Japan, 38, 3 (1968).

24.   E. Baltazzi, U. S. Pat. 3,343,941 (Sept. 26, 1967).

25.   A. A. Crafts, "The Chemistry and Mode of Action of
      Herbicides", Interscience Publishers, Inc., New
      York, 1961, p. 217.

26.   G. G. Allan, Belg. Pat. 706,509 (Dec. 15, 1967).

27. F. B. Folckemer, R. E. Hanson, and A. Miller, Belg.
     Pat. 648,606 (Nov. 30, 1964); U. S. Pat. 3,318,769
     (May 9, 1967).

28. Chem. Eng. News, 50 (23), 68 (1972).

29. G. G. Allan, C. S. Chopra, A. N. Neogi, and R. M.
     Wilkins, Nature, 234, 5328, 349 (1971).

30. G. G. Allan, et al., Chem. Tech., 4, 171 (1973).

31. I. Krisehenbaum, J. Polymer Sci., 3A, 1869 (1965).

32. R. Hill and E. E. Walker, J. Polymer Sci., 3, 614
     (1948).

33. T. F. Bradley and W. B. Johnston, Ind. Eng. Chem.,
     33, 86 (1941).

34. J. Crank, "Mathematics of Diffusion", Oxford
     University Press, London, 1956.

35. H. Fujita, "Diffusion in Polymers", edited by
     J. Crank and G. T. W. Park, Academic Press, New
     York, 89, 1968.

36. G. G. Allan and A. N. Neogi, Int. Pest. Control,
     July-Aug. (1972).

37. P. H. Terry and A. B. Borokovea, J. Med. Chem., 11,
     958 (1968).

38. G. G. Allan, C. S. Chopra, A. N. Neogi, and R. M.
     Wilkins, Tappi, 54, 1293 (1971).

39. A. N. Neogi, Ph.D. Thesis, University of Washington,
     1970.

40. R. M. Wilkins, M.S. Thesis, University of Washing-
     ton, 1969.

41. H. Morawetz and E. Gaetjens, J. Polymer Sci., 32,
     526 (1958).

42. R. P. Petri, Kunstoffe, 53, 421 (1963).

43. R. F. B. Davies and G. E. Reynolds, J. Appl. Polymer,
     Sci., 12, 47 (1968).

44. V. V. Dovlatyan and D. A. Kostanyan, Izv. Akad. Nauk. Arm. SSR. Khim. Nauk, 18 (3), 325 (1965).

45. J. H. Rediske and G. R. Staebler, Forest Sci., 8, 353 (1962).

46. G. G. Allan, C. S. Chopra, and R. M. Russel, Int. Pest. Control, March-April (1972).

47. R. M. Dourojianni, Agronomia (La Molina, Peru), 30 (1), 35 (1963).

48. J. Ramirez Sanchez, Boletin del Instituto Forestal Latino Americano de Investigacion y Capocitacion, 16, 54 (1964).

49. G. G. Allan, R. J. Gara, and R. M. Wilkins (in press).

50. G. G. Allan and A. N. Neogi, Int. Pest. Control, 14 (1972).

AUTHOR INDEX

Page numbers underlined are for the complete reference.

SUBJECT INDEX

231